PREFACE

We are in the throes of a health care system gone rogue. What should have been universal health care for everyone in 1965 covered only the elderly, and without drug coverage, due to a narrow political window. A promise was made then by Congress to finish the task of universal coverage at a later date. That time never arrived, in spite of passage of Part D drug coverage with the Medicare Modernization Act of 2003.

Richard Boudreau's timely probe into universal and single-payer health care is essential, especially with the upcoming presidential election; knowing the history of our attempts at health care reform, we can offer real and feasible solutions. We are in a perpetual health care crisis with ever increasing insurance premiums, deductibles, and co-pays and with more limited referral panels and other road-blocks to care. Health care is a human right, as adopted in 1948 by the United Nations General Assembly in its Universal Declaration of Human Rights.

The Clinton health care plan of 1993 was a fiasco. Five hundred prominent citizens, including clergy, were selected as delegates to discuss what would be the Hillary Plan. The government agenda was predetermined. The five hundred delegates were present at a sham discussion that was inconsequential in the final proposal. Even their reimbursements were delayed or denied. The truth came out later that the Hillary Plan was to be a giveaway to the largest health insurance providers, with consolidation leading to better government control of health care. Ironically, it was defeated after very contentious congressional discussion, but de novo consolidation did occur until it was preempted by the Affordable Care Act (ACA) of 2010.

The ACA failed to give universal coverage. It was not cost-effective. It relied too heavily on Medicaid, founded in 1965, which had never been successful due to chronic underfunding and limited participation by physicians. The political forces of our present conservative government have virtually dismantled the ACA. So what to do?

Boudreau has given us the historical insights and understanding of our early forays into health care. The stage is now set for a critical showdown in an attempt to resurrect our moribund health care system. Medical costs are unsustainable as two-thirds of bankruptcies come from medical expenses in spite of health insurance coverage. Drug prices, especially for cancer patients, have gone through the roof, costing upwards of $100,000 a year. There is a reality and value disconnect regarding the curative quality of the drugs, which may offer only a few months of a meaningful and sustainable life.

Medicare was created in 1965; its golden years followed, extending into the 1990s. Most recently, corporate America under government auspices has taken greater control over health care. The government mandate of the electronic health record (eHR) is more for billing than for patient care; eHRs do not generally interface with each other. President Obama could have given physicians a federal eHR already paid for with taxpayer monies. Instead, physicians searched for an eHR that fit their needs. New systems were not designed for the specific needs of the generalist and were too expensive. Many physicians with increasing practice expenses and diminishing reimbursements could not afford to stay in their practices, opting for early retirement or a corporate practice.

The present clinical approach adopted by medical schools emphasizes diagnosis by the test rather than the traditional initial history and physical. Present clinical histories are usually checklists filled out by the patient in private and not generally reviewed by the physician, who say, "We will perform the tests first, then decide what is your problem." The end result of innovation appears to be fragmented health care, requiring more referrals to more specialists as we are gifted with more sophisticated and expensive technology.

The technology developed by the pharmaceutical industry and by medical innovators with new diagnostics (radiologic and nuclear scans, laboratory tests) is more expensive than in any other country. Our government does not adequately protect the public from these usurious costs.

The physical examination is now generally briefer with the new technology. Presently, doctors cannot maintain eye contact with the patient because they are typing at a computer. The stethoscope, once the symbol of the physician, has become obsolete. Reliance on technology has taken precedence. Medical school professors are under the gun to produce evidence-based studies to develop more instruments, procedures, and medications to enhance the bottom line of the school or institution. The cycle of the present upward cost spiral must be given immediate attention.

Boudreau deftly presents the case for universal health care and a single-payer system to replace our tortured current one. The American public must be educated and urged to enter the discussion now, as we cannot trust politicians to lead us out of our medical morass. We must be prepared to enter the health care fray.

The fight is on.

Jerome P. Helman, MD
Board Certified in Internal Medicine and Gastroenterology
Adjunct Assistant Professor in the Providence John Wayne Cancer Institute

US UNIVERSAL
HEALTH CARE
◆◆◆ IN ◆◆◆
2020

RICHARD GEORGE BOUDREAU

Faculty, Loyola Marymount Univ. Bioethics Institute
Faculty, UCLA Dept. Oral and Maxillofacial Surgery

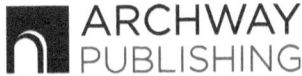

ARCHWAY
PUBLISHING

Archway Publishing books may be ordered through booksellers or by contacting:

Archway Publishing
1663 Liberty Drive
Bloomington, IN 47403
www.archwaypublishing.com
1 (888) 242-5904

ISBN: 978-1-4808-8326-0 (sc)
ISBN: 978-1-4808-8325-3 (hc)
ISBN: 978-1-4808-8327-7 (e)

Library of Congress Control Number: 2019914716

Print information available on the last page.

Archway Publishing rev. date: 9/23/2019

ABSTRACT

Healthcare in the United States is a multitrillion-dollar industry, consisting of many stakeholders from many different paths. The problem, however, is that while these stakeholders are dictating everything from healthcare delivery to payment, what they seem to forget about is the user of healthcare services: the patient. The problem is that healthcare costs in the United States are so out of control, it is difficult to see a way to rein them in. The Affordable Care Act, which passed in 2010, was to have been a comprehensive effort to guarantee coverage for all while reducing costs; unfortunately, because of many factors, the legislation has only succeeded partially in these goals. Furthermore, many continue to chip away at the legislation, bit by bit.

The reality of the situation here is that while most countries in the developed world consider health care a basic human right, the United States continues struggling with how to reduce costs, while ensuring that those who need health care can obtain it. In reality, promoting a Medicare for All agenda, even assuming it would pass Congress, make it to a president's desk, and be signed into legislation, would only solve part of the issue. It's nice to think of insurance for everyone. Just as important, though, is ensuring that everyone has access to quality health care.

The goal of this book is to introduce several concepts. First, why and how we got to where we are today, as the health care crisis we are dealing with didn't just happen overnight. Rather, it is the result of many different steps and decisions, made throughout history, that have brought us to this point.

Second, we'll take a close look at the history of health care in the United States as well as the history of health care insurance in this country, to develop a better understanding of the roots of the issue. For instance, at one time, insurance companies were charitable endeavors, rather than for-profit business centers; they were charged with providing coverage to their members, no matter how ill or how old. We'll also examine the role that politics has played in health care legislation (or lack thereof, as we will see).

We will then take a very close look at the introduction and passage of the Patient Protection and Affordable Care Act of 2010, the process it went through, and the somewhat painful aftermath. We'll also focus on the Republican Party's unsuccessful attempts to overturn the legislation. We will examine whether the Affordable Care Act actually lived up to its promises and hype. We'll also explain the various parameters of the US health care system, such as the reliance on employer-sponsored health care, and why the elderly and poor continue slipping through the cracks.

The focus will then turn to whether universal coverage and a single-payer system can work in the United States by examining what's already in existence here: Medicare and the Veterans Health Administration. We'll also examine how states have handled health care reform and discuss whether they've succeeded at it. We'll look at the advantages and disadvantages of systems of other countries.

We will focus on health care reform as a platform for the Democratic Party in the upcoming presidential election and examine the focus of several of the leading contenders for the nomination. We'll spend time on a platform introduced by Physicians for a National Health Program (PNHP), then follow that up with arguments supporting the concept of Medicare for All; passing such a program could be fraught with a variety of challenges, and we'll discuss what those challenges are). We will then focus on other aspects of health care that can be implemented, even while politicos continue arguing over the merits of various methods of health care reform.

We'll then conclude with some thoughts about the idea of reform. It won't be pretty. It will be messy, but it can be done, as long as the different stakeholders focus on common interests. While many writers have attempted to focus on one aspect concerning health care reform and the difficulties in reaching consensus, this book is dedicated to compiling the facts, analyzing them, and determining where we went wrong in the past, why it happened, and how we can address the issues moving forward. Only by understanding the many different aspects of the US health care system, both the positives and the negatives, can we hope to spearhead meaningful health care reform that improves patient outcomes, without forcing them into bankruptcy.

CONTENTS

INTRODUCTION

Health care is a multitrillion-dollar industry in the United States. The industry consists of a variety of stakeholders: providers, private insurance companies, pharmaceutical companies, government-run agencies, and state and federal regulators. These stakeholders dictate a great deal when it comes to health care delivery and payment, which is why the concept of health care reform in America is so difficult. But such reform is necessary.

Though the United States is one of the wealthiest nations in the world, the disparities in income are only surpassed by the inequalities in access to health care. As time has gone on, health care costs have continued increasing, even as income has not, meaning a certain percentage of the population either can't afford to pay for medical care or is woefully underinsured.

The close ties between the health care situation (many call it a crisis) and the fiscal health of the United States, as a whole, has led to many proposals, over the decades, to fix the system. Solutions have ranged from introducing universal health care to adapting the existing systems. The most recent effort, the Patient Protection and Affordable Care Act, was passed in 2010, with the goal of providing more coverage to more Americans, while lowering health care costs. As we'll see later on, the success of the ACA (also called "Obamacare") has been mixed, at best.

Very simply, while most countries in the developed world perceive health care as a basic human right, the United States has yet to determine a way of creating and funding a single-payer universal health care system that will address the inequalities that exist and provide a better option for preventative medicine, intervention medicine, and long-term care (LTC). America continues struggling with this issue, but not because there isn't willingness to change; there is. The problem is that with the current health care situation, there is no one overall solution to fix it. This is because there is no one issue to blame for where we are today.

Rather, today's system is the result of decades of decisions and actions from many stakeholders. While politicians and activists scream rhetoric in catchy phrases and one-liners ("Abolish Obamacare," "Medicare for All"), there is no simple one-source solution for this issue. Basically, until the history of health care in America (and the action of the industry's stakeholders, as well as their wants and needs) is fully understood, there can be no meaningful reform.

Fixing the current health care system requires addressing many factors, not just insurance coverage. Certainly, ensuring coverage for everyone in the United States and revamping the ACA are good starts. But they, in and of themselves, won't fix the problem. As such, the purpose of this book is to delve into the myriad issues that brought the US health care system to its current point, where we are today, and determine if there is any way to fix it with the current solutions being suggested, such as a single-payer system or universal health care.

The book will focus on the current level of expenditure on medical care, along with the lack of access to quality health care for many, even with the full implementation of the ACA. We'll also provide an honest assessment of health care in other Western industrialized nations, as well as examining examples of single-payer activities (Veterans Health Administration) and universal coverage (Medicare and Medicaid). We will focus on health care inequality, especially when it comes to access to some of the more vulnerable citizens, such as the lower middle class and elderly.

We'll also analyze whether a single-payer system and universal coverage can exist in the United States, given its history, culture, and beliefs. With this information in hand, we'll focus on the best options for improving issues such as affordability, access to care, long-term viability, and distribution of funding or services. The end result will be a book that presents the issues impacting US health care today and plausible approaches toward making it more affordable and effective for the population. However, before coming up with plausible solutions or suggestions to today's health care issues, it's first a good idea to have a thorough understanding of exactly what problems we are facing.

CHAPTER ONE: HOW WE GOT HERE

◆ **Overview: The Bitter Pill**

ACCORDING TO PORTER AND LEE (2013), THE CURRENT
structure of health care delivery in the United States, which has
been sustained for decades, has relied on the following mutually
reinforcing elements: organization by specialty, with independent
private-practice physicians.

In other words, the concept of holistic health care is prac-
tically nonexistent in this day and age; "quality," as measured by
process compliance, as opposed to actual health care outcomes.
Cost accounting is driven by charges as opposed to costs. As we'll
see later on, the charges are arbitrary, with little to no rhyme or
reason. Fee-for-service payments by specialty are rampant with
cross-subsidies. Health care delivery systems have service-line duplication and little to no integration.

This means, for example, that a patient being attended by several
doctors, in several specialties, is likely to undergo the same blood
test for each physician, rather than experiencing a single blood draw,

from which all doctors can study. Patient population fragmentation means health care providers don't have a critical mass of patients with a different medical condition that can be studied. This lack of critical mass makes it difficult to determine health care outcomes based on specific treatments. IT systems are siloed around specific medical specialties, rather than being inclusive. Because of this, a cardiologist caring for a patient might not have access to information collected and analyzed by a pulmonologist. This separation leads to duplication of effort, misunderstandings, and higher costs.

Repetition and duplication of effort are concepts that will be seen throughout this book. Furthermore, the result of the points above has led to a system that is "so resistant to change [it explains why] incremental steps have had little impact" (Porter and Lee 2013). Part of the problem with health care reform proposals and the bills that have passed is that they nibble at the edges of the problem, rather than slicing through the issue and offering some real solutions. Many of the proposals address only one or two aspects of the above, rather than taking the entirety of the situation into account.

The issue was fully brought into the public consciousness in 2013, when *Time* magazine published the eye-opening article "Bitter Pill: Why Medical Bills Are Killing Us." In this 25,000-word article, author Steven Brill focused on horrific stories about the US health care system and its exorbitant and seemingly arbitrary costs. A couple of examples he introduced included a twenty-one-thousand-dollar charge for an indigestion diagnosis, which probably could have been solved with a bottle of Pepto-Bismol, and a ninety-four-thousand-dollar bill for a bloody nose. The latter, which was the result of a fall, led to a six-hour wait in an emergency room and a lot of tests, according to

Emilia Gilbert, the patient who underwent both the wait and tests (Brill 2013).

Brill, who eventually turned his long-form article into a book, also focused on a seriously ill patient, Sean Recchi, who had been diagnosed with non-Hodgkin's lymphoma. Recchi and wife, Stephanie, flew to MD Anderson Cancer Center in Houston for treatment. MD Anderson is arguably one of the best cancer clinics in the nation, which is fine. However, the self-employed Sean and Stephanie were told that the estimated cost of Sean's initial visit—just to determine his treatment plan and nothing else—would be a whopping forty-eight-thousand-dollars, due in advance. A week later, the couple was charged an additional thirty-five-thousand-dollars so he could begin treatment. Even though the money was paid upfront (with help from the couple's parents), the patient, who was "sweating and shaking with chills and pains," according to Stephanie, was held for ninety minutes in a reception area until the hospital confirmed that the check cleared. Sean was eventually allowed to see a doctor, only after he advanced MD Anderson seventy-five hundred dollars from his credit card.

While this story was shocking enough, it isn't at all uncommon. Noted Brill, "The hospital says there was nothing unusual about how Sean was kept waiting." Furthermore, the MD Anderson communications manager indicated that asking for advance payment for health care services is common, even if that payment is eighty-three thousand dollars out of pocket, which is what Sean and Stephanie had to pay before this very sick man could begin treatment.

Brill then went through the Recchis' bill, line by line. One treatment was for the generic version of Tylenol; one pill was $1.50. "You can buy 100 of them on Amazon for $1.49, even without a hospital's purchasing power," Brill said. Other charges, such as blood draw ($36) and lab analysis ($23–$76), were also indicated on the charges; such draws and analysis were fairly frequent, perhaps above and beyond what was necessary. Brill also discovered other markups in the bill and pointed out that while MD Anderson is an official nonprofit unit of the University of Texas, it has revenues that are greater than "the cost of the world-class care it provides."

The Recchi example was just a sample of what Brill introduced throughout his article, but the intent was clear. Health care costs are out of whack, especially for the diseases that health care is supposed to treat. Brill further reinforced his article by introducing a concept known as the "charge master," an arbitrary price list that is not based on anything concrete. The charge master is every hospital's internal price list; in Brill's words, it has "no process, no rationale, behind the core document that is the basis for hundreds of billions of dollars in health care bills."

The difficulty with the charge master, Brill commented, is that none of the prices on the documents are consistent with those of any other hospital, "nor do they seem to be based on anything objective—like cost —that any hospital executive I spoke with was able to explain" (Brill 2013).

This means that two patients can have the exact same treatment in two different hospitals but can be charged vastly different rates, simply because there is no standardization when it comes to pricing. Perhaps the most eye-opening part of this article was Brill's comparison of procedures paid by Medicare, versus that paid by private insurance. Needless to say, the Medicare charges were much more reasonable because of the way this system is structured.

What about disputing the high-cost bills? Good luck with that. "Bitter Pill" painted a nightmare scenario of working men and women who attempted to argue with the hospital bills and their charges, all without help or hope. In fact, the above-mentioned Emilia Gilbert ended up taking her case to court, where she lost. The article, with its heart-rending stories and massive amounts of research, won Brill (and *Time*) a National Magazine Award.

A couple of years later, Brill himself ended up in the patient's position, with a bubble on his heart. The process, he said, helped him analyze health care, and the US health care system, from a patient's perspective, and first-hand. It was an eye-opener for him. Because most patients participating in the US health care system are emotional and fearful to begin with, the charges and confusion just add more emotion and fear to an already difficult situation. "A patient in the American health care system has very little leverage, has very little knowledge, has very little power," Brill told NPR during an interview in 2015. The problem is that, unlike Brill and others, many in the health care system might not know enough, or argue enough, against the charges. Nor has Brill been the only one to point fingers at the flawed situation that is the US health care system.

In her book, *An American Sickness: How Healthcare Became Big Business and How You Can Take It Back*, author Elisabeth Rosenthal shares the discussion she had with Stephen Parente, a health economist at the University of Minnesota and advisor to John McCain during the 2008 US presidential election. Parente told the author that many studies overstate excessive health care spending in the

United States. However, the situation became personal when his elderly mother was hospitalized. Parente's story was like those heard from many others: Dozens of doctors, sending separate bills, and his inability to decipher any of them clearly (Rosenthal 2018).

The bills all consisted of large numbers, while insurance paid only a tiny fraction of each bill (Rosenthal 2018). Parente said, in disgust, "Imagine if a home contractor worked this way. He estimates $125,000 for your kitchen, and then takes $10,000 when it's done. Would anyone ever renovate?" Rosenthal added, "In no other industry do prices for a product vary by a factor of ten, depending on where it is purchased, as is the case for bills I've seen for echocardiograms, MRI scans and blood tests to gauge thyroid function or vitamin D levels."

Rosenthal told the story of another patient, Jeffrey Kivi, who knew something about pharmaceutical prices. Before his job as a chemistry teacher at Stuyvesant High School in New York, he had been a researcher at Abbott Laboratories, so he knew something about drugs, their costs, and their manufacturing process. Kivi, who suffered from psoriatic arthritis, visited Beth Israel Hospital every six weeks, where he would receive an infusion of a drug called Remicade. Beth Israel was his outpatient clinic of choice, as his rheumatologist, Paula Rackoff, had her practice there. The treatment cost nineteen thousand dollars each visit, but Kivi had good insurance under Emblem Health and didn't worry about it.

In 2013, Rackoff moved her practice to NYU's Langone Medical Center; at first, this seemed to be ideal for Rackoff, as it was more convenient for him. Furthermore, the center was open nights and weekends, so he didn't have to take time off to get treatment. He expected he would have to pay a little more as the services, over-all, were somewhat better. However, the first treatment at the new hospital was billed at $98,575.98 and the second billing came in at $110,410.82. The third treatment, and additional treatments there-after, were billed at $132,791.04. "It was the same dose as always," Rosenthal said, "in the same form, prescribed by the same doctor" (Rosenthal 2018, p. 12).

When Kivi and Rosenberg both tried to get to the bottom of the reason why the mark-up was so much higher, an NYU patient-care representative said that, shipping costs, storage costs, and other ad-ministrative costs were the likely culprit. "In the end, she said that I should pay no attention to how much money my insurance company was being forced to pay. After all it's not costing me anything," Kivi told Rosenthal (p. 13).

When Rosenthal continued asking questions, she said the expla-nations became even less convincing. One such explanation, from the public affairs department, mentioned that Kivi was receiving aggressive treatments because he was a large man, and Remicade is dosed according to weight; the teacher was over six feet in height and weight nearly four hundred pounds. Even with all of this in mind, an independent researcher told Rosenberg that, even at a higher dosage, the cost per dosage should only have been $1,200, rather than the $132,000 that was being charged to Emblem Health.

One of Remicade's inventors, NYU professor Jan Vilcek, do-nated a share of his patent royalties to Langone Medical Center out of gratitude for helping him to re-establish his career in the United States (he was originally from Slovakia and had emigrated to America). NYU sold most of its rights to the royalties in 2007 for

$650 million but still receives payment, as long as profits from the drug increase above a particular financial bar that is undisclosed. "With charges like $132,000," Rosenthal commented, "chances are that bar will be crossed" (p. 13).

This likely explained why the NYU charges were higher than those from Beth Israel. What stunned Kivi, however, was that instead of attempting to secure a deep discount for payment, Emblem Health paid almost the entire amount, without any question or dispute. Basically, Emblem was paying $1 million a year to NYU Langone for these infusions. This meant that New York City residents were paying for part of that, with their tax dollars, as Kivi's insurance was through the public school at which he taught.

These and other stories prompted Rosenthal to outline the following "Economic Rules of the Dysfunctional Medical Market": More treatment is always better. Default to the most expensive option. A lifetime of treatment is preferable to a cure. As technologies age, prices can rise, rather than fall. There is no free choice. Patients are stuck. And they're stuck buying American. More competitors vying for business doesn't mean better prices; it can drive prices up, not down. Economies of scale don't translate to lower prices. With their market power, big providers can simply demand more. There is no such thing as a fixed price for a procedure or test. And the uninsured pay the highest prices of all. There are no standards for billing. There's money to be made in billing for anything and everything. Prices will rise to whatever the market will bear.

Rosenthal's book, and her viewpoint, involve more a call to arms for patients to take back their health care and to reduce costs. She also lauds health care in other countries as more effective and less expensive, which isn't quite true, as we will see later. She also tends to blame doctors for the high cost of health care; while this is true, to an extent, doctors and other health care providers are tired of dealing with the administrative burden that the US health care system puts on them. While Rosenthal's argument is flawed in some cases, she is correct that as health care in the United States currently stands, it is simply unsustainable.

Getting back to Brill, the reaction to his article and eventual book ranged from supportive to critical. However, Brill's and Rosenthal's contentions are that the US health care system, as it stands, is in a mess. "Unless you are protected by Medicare, the health care market is not a market at all. It's a crapshoot," Brill said. "People fare differently according to circumstances they can neither control nor predict." Furthermore, patients fare different, in terms of cost, from hospital to hospital, which can make comparison shopping for procedures very difficult.

◆ Focus on the Numbers

Health care prices are going up. There is no doubt about it. Singhal et al. (2018) point out that one reason for the increase is because demand is also rising. The population in the United States is growing older, and it is living longer. This means that "old-age" diseases that once were almost nonexistent, because people died earlier, are facts of life.

Older people are also searching for a better quality of life in their golden years. The problem, however, is that consumers, employers, and the government continue to see the financial burden of health care increase faster than incomes or revenue (Singhal, Latko, and Martin 2018). The concerns are well-founded. According to the Centers for Medicare & Medicaid Services (2018), US health care spending grew 3.9 percent in 2017, translating to $3.5 trillion, or $10,739 per person. From an economic perspective, health care spending accounted for a whopping 17.9 percent of the national GDP (National Health Expenditure Data—Historical 2018).

So health care costs in the United States are high and continue to increase. The scenario wouldn't be so bad, if the outcomes matched the amount spent. But a report from the Commonwealth Fund said that, while the United States spends more, per capita, than any other high-income country, the population, overall, has poorer health and lower life expectancies than the other nations (Schneider et al. 2017). When measured against ten other high-income countries, America ranked last in access, equity, and health care outcomes, and next-to-last in administrative efficiencies. This latter would likely not surprise many US health care providers.

Additionally, the United States ranked last on access to care and has the worst performance among other countries when it comes to affordability. The report led the Commonwealth Fund authors to note that "despite spending nearly twice as much as several other countries, the country's performance is lackluster." While the Affordable Care Act has improved some aspects of performance within the health care system, the report added, "the U.S. still greatly lags countries with universal insurance coverage."

Another report from the Harvard T.H. Chan School of Public Health agreed with the Commonwealth Fund's findings, adding that the 17.8 percent of US dollars directed toward health care was far higher than the 9.6 percent GDP paid in Australia and the 12.4 per-cent reported by Switzerland (Papanicolas, Woskie, and Jha 2018). Furthermore, the proportion of population in the United States with health insurance was 90 percent. Certainly, this shows that much of the population is covered. However, in comparison with other countries, the US average is very low; population coverage in other countries was 99 percent and above. And while the United States spends about twice as much as other high-income countries on medical care, utilization rates were "largely similar to those in other nations," according to a Harvard University report, which was written up in the *Journal of the American Medical Association*.

The report also found that the main drivers of the overall cost differences between US health care and that of the rest of the world included prices of labor and goods (specifically, pharmaceuticals), administrative costs, and the high salaries of health care providers, notably, physicians (Papanicolas, Woskie, and Jha 2018). Basically, doctors in the United States command higher salaries than their counterparts in Canada or Germany. Pharmaceutical costs, specifically, were noteworthy. Spending per capita for pharmaceuticals in the United States was $1,443, versus a range of $466–$939 in other countries.

Why, exactly, are American people paying more for health care? What follows are some answers: Prices for health care goods and services are higher in the United States than elsewhere (Frakt 2018). This is another point that will continue to be focused on: that health care costs are very much out of hand. Another point is that it has taken years to get to where we are today. Johns Hopkins professor Gerard Anderson noted that "the differential between what the U.S.

and other industrialized countries pay for prescriptions and for hospital and physician services continues to widen, over time."

Lack of competition in the American health care system. Though conservatives and others who are against a universal system claim that the United States has a free market when it comes to health care, this isn't true. As mentioned above, there is little consumer choice when it comes to selecting health care services; most Americans are required to select health care, based on what their insurance will and will not cover. Another issue is that in a free market, consumers have the ability to compare prices before selecting on a product or service. The fact that prices aren't standardized for procedures makes this very difficult. Additionally, consumers will go to hospitals and specialists through referrals from other health care providers, versus actual choice. And finally, periods of rapid growth in US health care spending have tended to coincide with rapid growth in health care price markups. Noted Frakt, "This is what one would expect in markets with low levels of competition." So, to repeat, the US health care system is not a free-market system.

Rising administrative costs. Billing and price negotiations across many third-party private payers could explain part of the issue. Furthermore, costs associated with many insurers, each requiring different types of billing documentation, could also be adding to the issue; one recent study points to the fact that the United States "has higher health care administrative costs than other wealthy countries," something already pointed out in this book. Princeton health economist Janet Curie noted, "We have big pharma vs. big insurance vs. big hospital networks," with patients, employers, and even the government paying the bills. Even large public health programs can't keep a lid on prices; for example, Medicare can't negotiate, as a whole, for drug prices. Unlike single-payer insurance, which offers a more standardized approach when it comes to payment, the patchwork quilt of private insurance companies, and what treatments they will and won't accept, adds stress to an already dysfunctional system.

Private insurance companies. The US health care system is in the grip of insurance companies. Rather than being an inactive participant in the process of health care delivery and access, as they are in other countries, such companies are the deciding factor as to who gets which treatment. More often than not, if a treatment isn't covered by insurance, a patient won't seek it. Commentator Nathan Sass, in his response to Brill's article/book, indicated that the cause of the overcharges mentioned in Brill's article wasn't so much actual health care prices, as much as it was due to insurance itself, rather than the lack of it (Sass 2013). Basically, the health care system means the providers are allowed to bill a third party (insurance companies), and the consumer doesn't know what is actually on the bill.

Sass pointed out, and quite rightly, that if 99 percent of patients were similar to those in Brill's case studies and directly billed for medical services, "wouldn't people tell them to go to hell, and go to a hospital that charges the $0.13 that the pill should actually cost?" Sass's conclusion: The system is broken because buyers and sellers don't discuss the price for a service, with the purchase being made anyway, and someone else picking up the tab. Getting more people on insurance, he pointed out, is making the problem worse, rather than solving it (Sass 2013). This was pointed out in the above study concerning Emblem Health and its acceptance of abnormally high charges for Remicade.

The physicians, themselves. We can discuss the high cost of doctors' salaries, but weighed against this are the high costs of medical schools that help lead to such high salaries. Medical students end up taking years to pay off debts, which also explains why more end up in higher-paying specialties than as general practitioners. Speaking of medical schools, doctors, for the most part, are rarely taught about the actual cost of health care (Rosenthal 2018). The ignorance ends up having an implication on both that physician's future practice and the patients who are being treated. "How can a doctor prescribe the best medicine for a patient if he or she doesn't know the relative costs of three classes of drugs?"

Furthermore, until about thirty years ago, the idea of practice management—that a physician should run his or her practice, more like a business with profits and losses—was looked down upon by many of the older doctors. These days, especially, cost and cost-effectiveness should be a part of medical school curricula, with national medical boards regularly testing this particular knowledge (Rosenthal 2018).

Opaque information. Individual doctors can have a difficult time obtaining prices for various procedures. This is because hospital finance departments and treatment centers keep those prices hidden. Again, the business side of health care is separated from the treatment side, which in turn breeds ignorance or indifference. Nor is it just the finance departments that put up roadblocks. The situation is further complicated by the fact that discounted contracted rates negotiated by the provider's financial departments with insurance companies are protected by nondisclosure agreements. While some states declared such gag clauses illegal, physicians can be afraid to divulge the information, or they could be hiding something that could make money for them.

Extraordinarily high drug costs. Big Pharma, as it is known, invests a great deal of money on research and trials of new drugs and cures. However, the industry has come a long way from Jonas Salk's comment in reference to a patent for his polio vaccine, which eliminated a horrible disease: "Well ... I would say, there is no patent. Could you patent the sun?" (Rosenberg 2018, p. 94). Fast-forward several decades, and the concept of legitimate intellectual property in medicine has changed. The average number of patents per drug was 2.5 in 1990; it rose to 3.5 by 2005 and has expanded since then. Many of today's best-selling medicines are covered by more than five patents, and some, by more than a dozen. These patents cover not only the molecules involved with the drug but the processes that create each formulation, as well as the delivery systems (e.g., special coatings over the pill).

To summarize everything above:

The United States has struggled to create and fund a single-payer system because of the many stakeholders involved with the industry. Hugely varying medical costs from treatment center to treatment center means a lack of price standardization. This, in turn, robs consumers of the ability to make an informed choice when it comes to selecting a medical procedure. While the United States spends a huge amount of its GDP on health care, patient outcomes are shown to be worse than those in other industrialized nations where health care expenditure is far less.

Private insurance companies, which play an active role in patient choice, can limit effective treatment. Medical schools, with their high costs, have led to high-salaried physicians, which is exacerbating the problem. Drug costs are also obscenely high, due to patent claims and many loopholes. The above explains, to an extent, why throwing legislation at the problem isn't working. The system is too vast and complex for new rules or regulations to be effective. So the question becomes, how did we get here in the first place? The answer lies with the history of US health care and the rise of the insurance industries.

CHAPTER TWO: DISSECTING THE HISTORY OF HEALTH CARE IN THE UNITED STATES

◆ **A History of Health Care**

TODAY'S HEALTH CARE SCENARIO AND WOES DIDN'T happen overnight. Rather, changes in health care delivery, and payment for services, changed and evolved incrementally, over decades.

Going back to the dawn of the twentieth century, a little more than a hundred years ago, the US medical care landscape was vastly different from what it is today; disease and death were the norm, rather than the exception. People regularly died from what today we consider preventable diseases. Professional physician services were inadequate in the preindustrial era, due to poor medical practices; primitive procedures; missing institutional core; unstable demand; and disorganization of medical education (Shi and Singh 1998). Noted Rosenberg, "A hundred years ago, medical treatments were basic, cheap and not terribly effective." Most patients were treated in their homes, the industry was virtually unregulated, and the few hospitals that existed provided only minimal care.

As the Industrial Revolution continued chugging forward, and technology helped improve technique and education in health care, illnesses became more treatable and lifespans increased. Elements that helped move this along included a focus on urbanization, science and technology, institutionalization, dependency, cohesiveness and organization, licensing and educational reform (Shi and Singh 1998). The economy was moving from agrarian to industrial, with more people leaving the farmlands for the city. As such, health care methods and deliveries had to change as well.

The American Medical Association was founded in the mid-1800s. By the early 1900s, it emerged as a group that would strengthen doctors, as a whole, although later on in the twentieth century, it stymied efforts at health care reform. In its earlier days, however, the AMA, combined with emergence of general hospitals, strengthened the professional sovereignty of doctors by encouraging a common interest among physicians, as well as affording them a "well-organized medical profession." Hospitals gave physicians a base from which to practice, while the AMA helped lead the push toward more organized medicine (Griffin 2017). By 1910, surgery was slowly being accepted as a common response to tumors and appendicitis (Moseley 2008). Cleanliness became more routine in hospitals and health care treatments, and health outcomes improved (Moseley 2008). The American College of Surgeons was formed in 1913, becoming the first body to accredit hospitals.

World War I saw great advances when it came to caring for the wounded on the battlefield; the X-ray machine, for example, was in wide use when it came to searching for bullets in soldiers' bodies. Antiseptics saw wider use in preventing infection, and anesthesia was used during surgery. Ambulances were also in wide use during the First World War, bringing the concept of mobility to medicine and medical treatments.

By the end of the war, families had more money to spend but had less room in their homes to care for sick family members, meaning more were being admitted to the growing number of hospitals. The result was that by the 1920s, health care was improved but cost more, due to growing demand and higher quality standards required for physicians and hospitals. By 1929, the average American family's medical expenses were $103, approximately 5 percent of the average annual income at the time.

With World War II came surgical specialization and the use of sulfonamides and, later on, penicillin to treat infections. Following the war, health care continued to improve. For example, materials such as plastics began being used for everything from heart valves to suture material, thus improving patients' chances for survival. Vaccines were introduced, leading to better outcomes for diseases such as polio, chicken pox, and measles. While the X-ray was a tool founded in the late nineteenth century, the advancement of imaging techniques in the twentieth century helped doctors find diseases, while more and more drugs were unveiled to help battle those diseases. In the latter half of the twentieth century, heart, lung, and kidney transplants become more routine, boosting survival rates that would have been unimaginable decades beforehand. Intensive care units in hospitals were staffed by those who understood critical care, which, in turn, led to higher recovery rates for patients.

This was the upside in medical technology. The downside is that these miracles increased the costs of medical care. While families could once pay for treatments out of pocket, doing so was becoming increasingly difficult. Health care insurance stepped up to help defray the costs of medicine.

◆ The Dawn and Implementation of Health Insurance

The US health care debate, and how such health care is supposed to be paid for, is considered a modern issue. Issues such as deductibles, co-pays, and premiums lead the national discourse. It's interesting to note that while claim forms and explanations of benefits are an integral part of the US health care system, none of this existed a century ago (Rosenberg 2018). Google the term "history of private insurance in the United States," and the general consensus is that health insurance, as we know it today, started in the 1920s. In truth, however, the health care insurance discussion stretches back more than a century and a half. One of the earliest health care proposals, at the federal level, was issued with the 1854 Bill for the Benefit of Indigent Insane (Manchikanti et al. 2017). And true to form, that bill created controversy and was ultimately vetoed by President Franklin Pierce; his argument was that the federal government shouldn't be committed to social welfare. A few decades later, the federal government did become involved in health care, when it established national medical care in the South, with construction of forty hospitals and employment of more than a hundred doctors after the Civil War.

In the meantime, the earliest health insurance policies were designed to compensate for lost income while workers were ill. Long absences were a problem for companies depending on manual labor.

They were also a problem for the workers. If they took days off due to illness, they weren't paid. As such, late-nineteenth-century employers often hired doctors to provide on-the-job care for workers. As medical treatments and knowledge improved in the early twentieth century, the concept of paying a set amount in advance for health care treatment, to prevent a larger bill down the road, evolved (Rosenthal 2018). In the early days, prepayment was informal; hospitals independently opted to provide services on a prepaid basis.

The model for today's insurance plans was developed at Baylor University Medical Center in Dallas (now Baylor Scott & White Health). At the time, as hospitals and physicians started charging more money for health care than people could legitimately afford, a group of teachers came together to create the Baylor University Hospital program, under the direction of Justin Ford Kimball, an administrator at the Dallas college (Griffin 2017; see also Blue Cross and Blue Shield Association History 1995). As part of the plan, the teachers agreed to prepay for future medical services, up to twenty-one days in advance. The idea was that for a set price per month, subscribers would pay into a fund that would, if needed, cover the full cost of hospitalization. Other Dallas employee groups joined the program, and it began attracting attention across the United States (Blue Cross and Blue Shield Association History 2014). Similar programs cropped up in Iowa and Illinois; these plans involved only one hospital, however (Blue Cross and Blue Shield Association History 2014).

The Blue Cross name and symbol were trademarked in 1934, and by 1935, fifteen Blue Cross plans existed in eleven states. The problem with this plan was that it covered only hospital services, not physician visits. To address this particular issue, a group of employers in the lumber and mining industries in the Northwest joined to provide physician services to employees. The first modern Blue Shield plan, as it was known, was established in 1939 in California (Blue Cross and Blue Shield Association History 2014). Based on the earlier programs, this plan allowed customers to receive physician services for $1.70 a month. Only those with incomes under three thousand dollars were eligible for the program. Medical societies in other states developed similar programs; by the mid-1940s, many of the plans combined forces into a national group called the Associated Medical Care Plans, which were overseen by the AMA. The group eventually became known as the Blue Shield Association, which merged with Blue Cross in 1948; however, they were blocked from doing so by the AMA on the grounds that such cooperation between hospitals and physicians might lead to restraint of trade. The Blues eventually did merge, in the early 1980s.

◆ From Charity to For-Profit

Meanwhile, while the United States was embroiled in World War II, the Blue Cross Plans were proliferating in an effort to protect patient savings and keep hospitals, as well as the charitable groups that funded them, afloat. Contract practice and prepaid group practices became the prototypes of today's managed care plans; with contract practice, control of excessive utilization and traditional fee-for-service formats were highly preferred, while prepaid group practices provided consumers with comprehensive coverage for one fee.

It's important to understand that in the early days, health

insurance was mainly a charitable endeavor. The Blues were non-profit agencies, with the goal of protecting individuals who needed health care rather than profit motives. But medicine soon became more expensive, as technologies were perfected and more people received medical care. This meant a high insurance demand. Private companies realized the profit that could be earned selling insurance directly to customers.

Employers began getting into the act during World War II, when the National War Labor Board froze salaries during the conflict. Employers then turned to other means to attract workers, offering health insurance benefits; in lieu of any salary increase, companies shouldered the cost of health care for their employees. This was the foundation of the employer-sponsored health insurance seen today.

More for-profit companies flooded the marketplace; these companies weren't encumbered by the Blues' charitable mission (Rosenthal 2018). They accepted only younger, healthier patients on whom they could make a profit; Aetna and Cigna both offered major medical coverage by 1951. Thanks to aggressive marketing and closer ties to business (as opposed to a focus on health care), for-profits slowly gained market share through the 1970s and 1980s, making it difficult for the nonprofit Blues to compete. At the time, the Blues charged everyone the same, no matter how sick or old. But the organization was no match against the for-profit insurance plans. In many states, local Blue Cross plans faced insolvency, prompting mergers and acquisitions between the plans. In an effort to remain relevant and profitable, the Blues finally allowed member plans to become for-profit, thus ending the charitable focus of the organization.

◆ Pharmaceutical Costs

One large issue that continues to be addressed to day is the out-rageous cost of pharmaceuticals. Yet it wasn't always that way. For instance, when Frederick Banting discovered insulin in 1923, he didn't put his name on the patent, believing it was unethical for a doctor to profit from something that would save lives (Belluz 2019). Furthermore, Banting's co-inventors, James Collip and Charles Best, sold the patent to the University of Toronto for a grand total of $1. As mentioned above, Jonas Salk, who succeeded in developing a polio vaccine, also refused to profit from the drug.

Fast-forwarding a century, things have changed. Drug prices are ridiculously high, as anyone who has tried to fill a prescription knows. Just how high was brought home in 2015, when the price of Daraprim, a sixty-two-year-old go-to drug for parasitic infections, increased almost overnight from $13.50 to $750 a pill (Pollack 2015). That price hike brought Martin Shkreli into the spotlight; Shkreli, who owned the company that had the Daraprim patent, was unapologetic about the 5,000 percent price hike. He actually flaunted the fact he could jack up the prices and faced a huge round of criticism for his attitude. Shkreli, classified as the "Pharma Bro," eventually ended up in prison for defrauding investors.

However, Daraprim was not the only drug that faced a huge price hike; many health care providers questioned the huge prices increases of older drugs, some of them generic, which are often used for treatments. An article in the New York Times suggested that while some price increases were due to drug shortages, others were the result of a business strategy, involving the purchase of older, more neglected drugs and turning them into high-priced specialty drugs. Another example: Antibiotic drug Doxycycline went from $20 a bottle in October 2013 to $1,849 a bottle by April 2014.

Outrageously high pharmaceutical prices occur because in the United States, a lax regulatory environment encourages those high prices. In other countries, where governments exert much higher influence and controls over the entire health care process, this isn't the case. Another reason involves drug patents, which consist of a series of complex, tangled regulations involving which company owns which patent on which product.

For her part, Rosenberg (2018) blames the patent explosion, in part, on "perverse unintended consequences" of a well-intentioned piece of legislation, known as the Drug Price Competition and Patent Restoration Act of 1984. An amendment to the Food, Drug and Cosmetic Act passed in 1984, the gist of Hatch-Waxman, as it was called, was to help clarify the length and extent of patent protections on drugs, while offering generic drug manufacturers financial incentives to introduce cheaper versions to the market the moment the patents expired. Because Hatch-Waxman didn't require generic manufacturers to conduct fresh clinical trials before releasing their drugs, something had to be given to the original pharmaceutical patent-holders, and this involved a variety of new ways for those companies to actually extend their patents.

While Hatch-Waxman attempted to pinpoint when it would be fair business practice for generic manufacturers to issue their products, it instead gave brand makers a new ability to claim extended patent protection. The result is an "era in which multimillion-dollar court battles over patents [delayed] each generic entry, driving prices up in the process."

While the Generic Drug Enforcement Act of 1992 attempted to address the issue, it didn't help all that much. Adding insult to injury is that the actual character of inventing drugs and pharmaceuticals has changed. At one time, people running pharmaceutical companies were interested as much in social impact as in money. Industry executives came from respected academies, and research was focused on medical needs. These days, research decisions are based more on profit than on medical need.

◆ Health Care Insurance: A Political Football

While the Blues were creating nationwide programs for hospital and physician insurance, medical costs continued increasing. During the Great Depression of the 1930s, the health care discussion became heated at the federal level. High unemployment ended up creating the perfect climate for compulsory, universal health care, funded by the government. But the 1930s was not the first time the federal government attempted to deal with health insurance and medical care payments.

The first efforts focused on insurance were made in the late 1800s, during the Industrial Revolution (Griffin 2017). At that time, unions also became stronger; in an effort to shield members from catastrophic financial losses due to injury or illnesses, "sickness protection" came into being. At the time, there wasn't an organized, national structure, with much of this protection involving trial and error.

During the first decade of the twentieth century, the American working class wasn't supportive of the idea of compulsory health care; there wasn't much groundswell for such protection, the types that leading European nations would see as the century moved along. As such, while Theodore Roosevelt, the twenty-seventh president of the United States, advocated for health insurance, he didn't lead the charge, which came from nongovernmental organizations.

One such organization, the American Association of Labor Legislation (AAAL), drafted legislation targeting both the working class and low-income citizens. Under the proposed bill, qualified recipients would receive sick pay, maternity benefits, and a death benefit of fifty dollars to cover funeral expenses; the cost of such benefits would be split among states, employers, and employees.

While the AMA initially supported the bill, some of the local medical societies protested, citing concerns about physician compensation. The unions also had a problem with the bill, believing that compulsory health insurance would weaken their stance; a portion of their power, at the time, came from negotiating insurance benefits for union members. The AMA ultimately backed off and pulled support for the AALL bill. In the end, the AALL bill was unable to garner enough support to move forward.

After the start of World War I, Congress passed the War Risk Insurance Act to cover military personnel for death or injury; the act was later amended to extend financial support to dependents of those who served. While the War Risk insurance program ended with the conclusion of the war in 1918, benefits continued to be paid to survivors and their families.

Fast-forwarding to the 1930s, President Franklin Roosevelt

recognized the need to promote legislation to assist the elderly, especially during economically bad times. He also realized health care coverage was a huge issue, especially among older people, and worked on a bill that included old-age benefits, including medical benefits. But the AMA opposed a national health system, again citing concerns about how it would negatively impact its membership, the doctors. The end result was that any kind of benefits to the elderly would have to exclude a national health insurance program. Basically, FDR had to drop the health care coverage to pass the Social Security Act of 1935.

While the bill led to a system of old-age benefits, allowing states to create provisions for people who were unemployed, disabled, or both, there was no health care coverage involved as part of the act. As an aside, it's interesting to note that FDR, the Democratic president, opted not to include universal health care in the bill, especially in light of the fact that both houses of Congress, at the time, had Democratic majorities. Yale political science professor Jacob Hacker pointed out two reasons why health care reform was so difficult to pass under FDR: 1) Americans were distrustful of government, and 2) fragmented political institutions made transformative policies difficult to enact, especially when opposed by powerful interest groups (Hacker 2018). Despite the strength of his party behind him, FDR realized physician opposition would kill the bill if it included a national health insurance option.

With World War II on the horizon (pushed forward by the 1941 attack on Pearl Harbor), the nation's agenda shifted away from domestic issues to the upcoming conflict. As mentioned above, private insurance saw an uptick, as companies sought to attract talent through means other than increased salaries. Rather than moving toward a nationalized health care plan, unions, corporations, and private insurance companies began stepping into the breach to offer their own plans and assistance: the forerunner of private insurance.

Still, this didn't prevent legislators from continuing to try to focus on a nationalized health care plan. In an attempt to help the elderly and poor, the Wagner-Murray-Dingell Bill was introduced in 1943. It proposed universal health care, funded through a payroll tax; unsurprisingly, the bill was faced with intense opposition and eventually died in committee.

The next push toward nationalized health insurance came from President Harry S Truman, after World War II (Hansler 2017; see also Griffin 2017). Truman's plan included all Americans, rather than just the working class and poor citizens who had a hard time with affording health care. The reactions from Congress were mixed; some called the plan "socialist," noting that it came straight out of the Soviet Union, which added to the Red Scare that was facing the nation. Unsurprisingly, the AMA took a hard stance against the bill and introduced its own plan, which proposed private insurance options.

Furthermore, efforts to mandate state-sponsored health care likewise failed. In 1944, California Governor Earl Warren planned to introduce compulsory health insurance in the state, paid through Social Security (Merelli 2017). However, Campaigns Inc., founded by Clem Whitaker and Leone Baxter, teamed with the California Medical Association to oppose the plan and lobbied newspapers and the population against government intervention in health care. They even went so far as to note that "socialized medicine" was a German invention, which strummed an emotional chord, while American soldiers were fighting those same soldiers abroad.

Campaigns Inc. used a similar strategy some years later (on behalf of the American Medical Association) when President Truman attempted to introduce a public health plan. This time, Campaigns Inc. used anti-communist sentiment to strike fear in people about the specter of "socialized medicine," while putting a positive spin on the advantages of private practice medicine over the state-sponsored medical systems. This turned popular support against the Truman plan.

By the 1950s, the majority of working-age Americans obtained their health insurance through their jobs. While national health insurance was tabled during the early 1950s due to the Korean War, medicine was moving forward by leaps and bounds. Penicillin, discovered in the 1940s, became the first effective antibiotic, and in 1952, Jonas Salk's team at the University of Pittsburg created an effective polio vaccine, which was ultimately approved in 1955. At the same time, the first organ transplant was performed when Dr. Joseph Murray and Dr. David Hume removed a kidney from one man and successfully placed it in the man's twin brother. While such advancements in medicine were great, they came at a cost; during the 1950s, the cost of hospital care doubled, though little changed in the health insurance landscape.

Insurance and medical advances were a boon to those who were employed. However, while such benefits provided help to many, it did leave out vulnerable groups: those who were retired, the unemployed, those unable to work due to disability, and those with employers that didn't offer health insurance.

By 1960, the US government began tracking national health expenditures (NHE), calculating them as a percentage of the GDP. At the beginning of the decade, NHE account for 5 percent of GDP (ten years later, that figure almost doubled). In 1962, when John F. Kennedy was sworn in as the thirty-fifth president of the United States, he focused on a health care plan for senior citizens. He urged Americans to become involved in the legislative process and pushed Congress to pass his bill; it failed, however, against AMA opposition and fears of socialized medicine.

After Kennedy was assassinated in 1963, President Lyndon B. Johnson took up the health care cry, proposing an extension and expansion of the Social Security Act of 1935. Johnson's plan would ensure that senior and disabled citizens could access affordable health care through physicians and hospitals. But like his predecessors, Johnson found that implementing health care ideals was nothing short of impossible. In 1965, he signed into law the Social Security Amendments, which established the Medicare and Medicaid programs. Johnson faced stiff opposition to any kind of nationalized health care reform.

Julian Zelizer, author of *The Fierce Urgency of Now: Lyndon Johnson, Congress, and the Battle for the Great Society*, noted that doctors mounted a fierce lobbying blitz against the bill.   Additionally, the Southern Democrats, who controlled the committees at the time, didn't want the bill, either. It was only when the tides turned during the 1964 elections and Democrats regained control of Congress that the bill passed, but without the nationalized health care for all.

It's worth noting that Medicare, which is accepted today as a benefit for the elderly, is no longer the hot potato it was in the 1960s.

However, one way political operatives drag their opponents through the mud is by threatening Medicare. Those vague threats are enough to encourage Medicare beneficiaries to vote a specific way, one example of how health care reform is so highly politicized.

By 1970, NHE accounted for 6.9 percent of GDP, which was due, in part, to unexpectedly high Medicare expenses. Part of the problem, it seemed, was that the United States had not formalized a health insurance system; as a result, few had any idea how much it would cost to provide health care for an entire group of people. Still, the increase in NHE prompted yet another president—Richard Nixon—to try his own hand at a health care plan; given this was taking place on the heels of Medicare passage, members of Congress also worked on a plan. The Nixon plan's focus was that of employers offering health insurance to employees and even providing subsidies to those who had trouble affording the cost. The idea here was that the majority of Americans would have insurance through their employers and then be eligible for Medicare benefits when they retired.

Lawmakers felt the bill would satisfy the AMA, as doctors' fees and decisions wouldn't be influenced by government. Nixon and Massachusetts Senator Ted Kennedy, a Democrat, worked on the plan together under the spirit of bipartisanship. But Kennedy caved under pressure from the unions in a decision he later said was one of the largest mistakes of his life. Meanwhile, Nixon was able to expand Medicare through the Social Security Amendment of 1972 and the Health Maintenance Organization Act of 1973: a small victory, on which he planned to follow up. Then came the Watergate scandal, with the result being that support for Nixon's health care plan disappeared.

Anything having to do with Nixon was considered tainted, including health care reform. As such, when Nixon's vice president Gerald Ford took over the presidency, Ford did what he could to distance himself from the scandal, which included tabling health care reform. The end result was a health care industry that was considered in crisis by the end of the 1970s, aided by an economy suffering from heavy inflation and a recession. This was a dark period of US history and definitely not the time to introduce yet another effort toward a nationalized health care system.

◆ The 1980s: The Turning Point

While the NHE was on the rise for much of the middle part of the twentieth century, health care costs in the United States were manageable, political rhetoric aside. By 1980, "America was in the realm of other countries in per-capita health spending" (Frakt 2018). Yet during the decade, health spending began to skyrocket and become unmanageable for many families.

Some have blamed the deregulation policies of President Ronald Reagan for the shift, with the idea that a deregulated private insurance marketed spurred higher prices among companies. In 1986, Reagan signed the Consolidated Omnibus Budget Reconciliation Act, or COBRA, which meant former employees could continue to be enrolled in their previous employers' group health plan, as long as they agreed to pay the full premium (employer portion and employee contribution). However, that full premium was difficult for families to manage, especially those who didn't have full-time jobs. In addition, experts also point to the following reasons for the skyrocketing costs:

Late 1970s inflation. As mentioned above, the US economy was hurting during the late 1970s. High inflation was occurring due to high energy prices and low supply. Consumer confidence was also at a low. The United States was not a stranger to inflation, but it couldn't deal with high inflation. While other countries had more control systems when it came to inflation, the United States did not. The end result was that once spending constraints eased, suppliers of medical equipment ended up marketing costly technology innovations, finding customers in hospitals, medical practices, and elsewhere, "keeping up with rivals in the medical arms race," according to Henry Aaron, a Brookings Institution health economist. While increases in medical technologies and new drugs have been valuable and certainly helpful when it comes to reducing disease and increasing longevity, those innovations and technology have come at a high price.

Changes in payments to hospitals and doctors. Before the early 1980s, payments by insurers and Medicare were generally tied to costs (Frakt, *Medical Mystery: Something Happened to U.S. Health Spending after 1980*, 2018). For example, if a patient's surgery cost five thousand dollars, that's what the hospital was paid, plus a little more for reasonable profit. There wasn't any kind of mysterious spending or costs coming out of nowhere. However, payers began shifting financial risk to hospitals and doctors, thanks to a 1983 law. The law in question dictated that Medicare pay hospitals a fixed price per visit, regardless of actual costs. The legislation focused on diagnostic-related groups (DRGs), which mandated that hospitals be paid a fixed sum, per case, according to specific diagnoses. This meant that if providers could substantially reduce costs, they could earn a profit. If not, they lost money.

It's been surmised that hospitals have attempted to compensate for the lower government payments by charging privately insured patients higher rates, a practice known as cost-shifting (Altman 2012). The overall result of that legislation is that hospitals went from deliverers of health care to businesses that found themselves in the position of having to earn profits. The issue was exacerbated in the following decades, as medicine became less about patient health and wellness, and more about profits, shareholder confidence, and maintaining a healthy bottom line, rather than focusing on ensuring a healthy patient population.

◆ The Managed Care Debacle

While managed care actually got its start in the late nineteenth century, it emerged in the late 1980s and early 1990s as a way to allocate care, to reduce unneeded services, and to restrain costs, which were becoming unsustainable (Mechanic 2004). As early as the 1970s, the federal government began encouraging and subsidizing the growth of health-maintenance organizations (HMOs), which were prepaid group practices different from independent physician associations. The idea behind HMOs was that a primary care physician would direct health care for a patient and, if necessary, refer patients to specialists within that organization.

In theory, it was an ideal solution, as it would keep administrative costs within the same organization, thus lowering overall health care costs. However, because the prepaid group practices required a substantial amount of capital and organizational skills, financial structures began overshadowing the nonprofit HMO group model.

Furthermore, patient backlash began against the HMOs, due to the fact that they were restricted to visit certain health care providers and could only visit others on referrals. Dissatisfaction with HMOs led to other options: preferred provider organizations (PPOs) and point-of-service (POS) options. Under these plans, patients could see their own doctors but at a greater out-of-pocket expense.

Physicians were also against the managed care model, feeling it restricted them in terms of how to care for patients. Then came the horror stories about rationed health care, though in reality, actual instances of rationing were nonexistent. Still, other stories about patients being kicked out of hospitals before they were ready (health-wise) to be discharged, and an increasing wait to seek out specialized care, seemed to be a common theme within the strictly managed care system. Furthermore, the dilution of managed care to include patient choice ended up boosting costs and premiums; while the managed care of the 1980s–1990s did temporarily contain costs, that containment didn't last long.

◆ Clinton's Health Security Act

With the 1980s seeing a large increase in health care costs, Bill Clinton, Democrat candidate for the presidency, gave a speech before Congress in September 1992, calling for "America to fix a health care system that is badly broken" and to ensure that every American had access to health care (Skocpol 1995). When Clinton was elected, he had every reason to believe he had a mandate, especially when it came to health care reform. By 1990, public support for national health care reform was at an all-time high. Health care financing was a middle-class issue, as well as one for the working poor, with "bold health reform proposals" proliferating both inside and outside of government. The general public was fed up with the higher price of medical care and wanted something to be done about it.

Furthermore, the American Medical Association, typically the enemy of government-funded health care, developed a plan for guaranteed universal health insurance. Clinton's proposed "competition in a budget" seemed to satisfy the public's desire for universal and affordable coverage, while promoting cost reductions. In fact, it's safe to say that in addition to his campaign slogan "It's the economy, stupid," Clinton was elected president because of promises he made to reform health care and bring costs in line.

Once in office, Clinton got to work, hammering out a likely bill with the Democrat-controlled Congress known as the Health Security Act of 1993. This bill offered universal coverage while respecting the private insurance system; individuals could purchase insurance through state-based cooperatives, and companies couldn't deny anyone insurance based on preexisting conditions. Furthermore, employers would be required, by law, to offer health insurance to full-time employees. It was felt that even though employer-mandated insurance was part of the bill, the overall approach would please large employers and insurance companies.

As part of the proposed act, Clinton convened a task force under the leadership of Ira Magaziner and First Lady Hillary Clinton. Mrs. Clinton testified before the House Committee on Ways and Means and several other congressional committees (Hansler 2017). Later in 1993, the Health Security Act was introduced to Congress but failed to even make it to a floor vote. While health care reform was one reason why Clinton was elected, the health plan died, without a whimper.

◆ What Happened?

There were many reasons why the act failed to garner enough votes to even make it out of committee to a floor vote. Timing was one reason, while partisanship was another (Clymer, Pear, and Toner 1994). On the timing side, the task force conducted most of its work from January to May 1993, but the report couldn't be finalized until the president got his first budget through Congress, which didn't take place until the end of summer of 1993. Too much time passed between the introduction of the Health Security Act and it actually making it to Congress, meaning much of the momentum for pushing it forward died. Furthermore, while the task force did tap into participation from government officials, health policy experts, and state-level officials, other groups with a stake in the existing US health care system weren't officially represented (though the task force did consult with representatives of stakeholder groups). The fact that actual medical personnel weren't part of the deliberation did put some noises out of joint.

Another problem with the process was that the task force remained confidential during its deliberations, shrouding everything in mystery. As such, when the final plan was released, the public failed to have a good understanding of it, further eroding support for the legislation. Added to that, an alleged overreliance on governmental bureaucracy became an added liability to getting the proposed legislation passed.

Perhaps just as importantly, experts noted that the Clintons misread the political mandate. Certainly, the general population wanted health care reform. However, "they wanted something easy to understand, something that did not look as threatening as the Clinton plan," said Harvard School of Public Health scholar Bob Blendon. Adding to the din were lobbyists against the legislation, with more than $50 million put into advertising, "most by opponents and much of it simply false."

Then, there were the employers themselves, who struggled with the plan. Corporations were certainly interested in anything that would reduce their health care costs. But many executives were perplexed by the thousand-page-long Clinton plan, as well as "the expansion of Federal authority that Mr. Clinton was proposing." Corporate executives feared losing the right to tailor health care benefits to their employees' needs (Clymer, Pear, and Toner 1994). Concerns also existed among the Clinton plan's supporters, not the least of which was physicians objecting to proposed cutbacks in Medicare, and the unions' concerns that benefits won in collective bargaining would be taxed as part of the legislation.

To summarize, the plan took too long to make it to Congress (thus losing momentum), it was unwieldy and confusing, and groups from unions, to employers, to physicians found fault with it, based on their own special interests. In addition, and just as important, "the Clinton plan promised too much cost-cutting regulation and not enough payoffs to organized groups and middle-class citizens pleasantly ensconced in the existing U.S. health care system." Clinton had less of a mandate for health care reform than he thought.

It was no wonder that the legislation, beset with controversy and confusion as it was, didn't make it out of committee. So while Americans were for health care reform, they weren't for the disruption that was likely to come with it. This aspect, incidentally, is one reason why health care reform has been so difficult to put into place in a reasonable fashion. Still, not all was lost when it came to health care reform during the Clinton presidency. He did sign the Health Insurance Portability and Accountability Act of 1996, which established privacy standards and guaranteed that patients could have access to their health care records. It also placed restrictions on how preexisting conditions would be treated in group health plans.

In addition, as part of the Balanced Budget Act of 1997, the Children's Health Insurance Program (CHIP) expanded Medicaid assistance to uninsured children up to age nineteen, in families with incomes too high to qualify them for Medicaid. As such, the Clinton plans helped reduce costs affiliated with health care. However, and once again, the legislation only nibbled at the edges of the problem. It wasn't until Barack Obama made affordable care for all a centerpiece of his presidential campaign that the issue of health care moved forward in a dramatic fashion.

CHAPTER THREE: THE AFFORDABLE CARE ACT

◆ **The Legislation**

THE AFFORDABLE CARE ACT WE KNOW TODAY (ALSO known as Obamacare) was actually made up of two different bills (Boudreau 2017). H.R. 3962, the Affordable Health Care for America Act, and H.R. 3590, the Patient Protection and Affordable Care Act, were two segments of the process of creating the final revised Health Care and Education Affordability Act of 2010. Beginning in October 2009, H.R. 3962 was debated in the House of Representatives, and the Senate debated H.R. 3590. In the end, the House decided to focus on a revised version of the Senate bill, giving up on H.R. 3962 in favor of a changed version of H.R. 3590. These two pieces of legislation were created to address the issue of health care reform and the need for manageable methods for ensuring health insurance coverage for large segments of the adult population currently uninsured or underinsured. The progression of the legislative process and the addition of education funding stipulations in the final legislation show how complex the process is of getting legislation passed.

Michigan Democrat John Dingell introduced H.R. 3962 as a means of adopting changes to the current health insurance and health care payment systems to increase access to underserved populations and improve access to care. After being introduced in the House of Representatives in October 2009, it was sent to a variety of committees for assessment. Between October 29, 2009, and November 7, 2009, the bill was reviewed, amended, and reevaluated, including the addition of the Stupak-Pitts Amendment, which prohibited the use of abortion services for individuals receiving health insurance through public subsidies. This amendment led to controversies both in the signing of the initial House bill and later in the decisions made surrounding the passage of the amended Senate bill. In a close House vote, the amended H.R. 3962, which included the Stupak-Pitts Amendment, was passed by the House.

There were several basic aspects of H.R. 3962: health insurance market reforms, the creation of a Health Insurance Exchange, the introduction of a new public health insurance option overseen by the secretary of the Department of Health and Human Services, introducing an individual mandate, outlining specific employer benefits, defining methods for subsidizing premiums, the expansion of long-term insurance planning, prevention and wellness options, and the creation of a directive for advanced care planning. The bill also focused on methods for overseeing the application of the law and for improving methods for advancing individual care, including quality improvement initiatives, physician quality reporting, and fraud services.

One of the major provisions of H.R. 3962 was the creation of new standards in federal health insurance, in relation to both individual and small group markets, including banning efforts by insurance companies to prevent coverage for preexisting conditions and restricting the level of insurance that could be issued or the renewability of insurance policies based on health conditions (AMA 2009). The bill did allow for variations in premiums to be made based on some federal standards related to geographic location, age, and the size of the insured's family.

One of the more significant measures was to prohibit insurance companies from creating annual or lifetime limits that would prevent coverage for specific health conditions, including those that required long-term and end-of-life care. Other important measures in relation to the health insurance market included allowing students to stay on their parents' insurance policies longer and allowing for plans to be offered and sold across state lines.

The focus on prevention and wellness services was also a valuable component of this initial bill because it provided a means of creating incentives in small businesses to improving wellness programming in the workplace setting. In order to apply all the segments of the bill, the bill's authors also outlined grievance procedures and methods for addressing fraud and abuse, especially in relation to enrollment, affiliations, and the intent of new standards.

In September 2009, Representative Charles Rangel of New York introduced H.R. 3590 to the House of Representatives; it was passed the following month. Once in the Senate, though, this legislation went through a number of revisions, linked to revisions made to H.R. 3962. This revised bill was approved in March of 2010 and signed by the president on March 23, 2010, and enacted into law as the Health Care and Education Affordability Act of 2010. There were some significant differences among the first version of the House bill, the corresponding measures in H.R. 3962, and the end product.

Some of the changes that were adopted include a provision allowing insurers to increase premiums based on community ratings and tobacco use, rather than preexisting conditions. The provisions for health care coverage and the mandate for individuals was essentially the same between the two laws, though the enacted law focused on the continued use of a parent's policy for adult children up to the age of twenty-six. Both pieces of legislation focused on methods to subsidize the insurance of small companies (those with fewer than twenty-five employees), though minor differences existed in relation to the gross average income of those in small companies.

Federal subsidies were included in both acts, including a transition in the method for subsidizing Medicaid for adults and in the approach for purchasing health insurance across state borders. Perhaps the most controversial issue, that of the payment of abortion services, was also addressed in the amendments to the first piece of legislation and in the final; the Stupak-Pitts Amendment was excluded from the final draft of the bill in order to ensure passage.

The arguments against these health reform bills came from two specific groups: insurers, who feared the extensive reform measures would be costly, and Republican leaders, many of whom maintained that the health reform measures would require additional taxation and increase the deficit. Specifically, the law required that health insurers implemented minimum standards for health insurance policies and subsequently took away any caps that had been created to reduce the payment for large-scale or long-duration treatments.

Coverage caps, then, were essentially removed, requiring

insurers to pay a much higher price for people with long-term illnesses or expensive treatments. The law also focused on health insurance benefits for those with preexisting conditions, which again did
not allow insurers to place restrictions on those who could receive
coverage. These insurers, then, had a lot to lose with the passage of
this legislation and so sought methods to deter the passage through
the use of lobbying and other methods for getting their message
across.

One of these methods was to focus on the costs and economics
of health care reform, supporting the message that reform would
be costly, would result in additional taxation, and could possibly be
detrimental to many health insurance providers. Specific problems
that were the focus of health insurers included the call for refraining
from requiring co-payments for preventative health services and the
costs involved in treating individuals with long-term care needs and
preexisting conditions. Proponents of the bill maintained that cost
savings could be realized on a national level, rather than additional
expenditures, and that these related to everything from reduced reliance on public health insurance resources to fees provided to health
insurers and a broadened Medicare tax base, all of which promoted
a positive economic image of the act.

The intention of these bills and the final act were considered
positive; they linked some of the widespread issues in this country,
including lost productivity, lost employment, and low-income status,
to issues related to health care and wellness. The purpose was to find
a happy medium between the kind of national health coverage used
in most developed countries throughout the world and the use of a
private health insurance scenario that would address the needs of a

large population of underserved Americans. The bill demonstrated the necessity for compromise; it clearly did not meet all the original goals in relation to finding the best approaches to national health improvements, but it also addressed some of the major issues facing a large segment of the adult population.

H.R. 3962, the Affordable Health Care for America Act, and H.R. 3590, the Patient Protection and Affordable Care Act, led to the creation of the final Health Care and Education Affordability Act of 2010. Initially, developers sought to implement a plan that mirrored some of the sentiments regarding a national health program that had been promised under the Clinton administration and later embraced during Obama's campaign. While the bill did not completely accomplish the effort to provide a broad range of health care options for all citizens, it did serve as a means of compromise, advancing efforts to increase access to both health care and preventative care services for the underinsured and underserved nationwide.

Still, passage of the legislation wasn't easy, nor was it a foregone conclusion. For instance, in August 2009, as members of Congress returned to their districts and attended town hall meetings in attempts to discuss the legislation with their constituents, opposition to the efforts arose. Fears included a government takeover of the health care industry (Levy 2019). Stoking that unease were the so-called (and totally false) "death panels" that would withhold care from critically ill people. The panels were little more than end-of-life consults for those who were terminally ill, but opponents of the bill did what they could to spread misinformation (that end-of-life consult provision was dropped from the final legislation).

As the bill made its way through Congress, it seemed as though more compromises would need to be made. One example was that, in the House version, some representatives were leery of passing the bill, due to vague language concerning federal coverage of abortion. Throughout the process, in fact, abortion threatened to derail the legislation.

Adding to the problem was that the ACA was challenged by attorneys general in more than a dozen states. The concerns were that the individual mandate (requiring that most Americans carry health insurance or pay a penalty) was unconstitutional. Though many of the lawsuits were dismissed, beginning in late 2010, some federal judges ruled that the individual mandate exceeded the authority granted by the commerce clause and general welfare clause. The individual mandate was eventually struck from the legislation when President Donald Trump took office, with help from the Republican-controlled Congress.

The framers of the ACA attempted to put a damper on insurers' profits and executives' salaries by requiring them to spend 80 to 85 percent on every premium dollar on patient care (Rosenthal 2017). Unsurprisingly, insurers fought against this provision. What's ironic is that Medicare uses 98 percent of its funding for health care and only 2 percent for administration. Nor did the rancor end with the bill's signing. Following the 2010 midterm elections, Republicans (who had pledged to repeal the health care bill), gained control of the House of Representatives. The repeal, however, failed in the Democrat-controlled Senate. Other similar repeals continued to fail.

◆ The Aftermath of the ACA

The ACA was implemented in 2014, bringing with it the individual mandate, subsidized marketplace coverage, and state Medicaid expansions (Courtemanche et al. 2018). However, not all states agreed to expand Medicaid coverage under the ACA; this ended up leaving many, especially lower-income individuals, without affordable coverage. The Medicaid expansion was originally meant to be national; however, a June 2012 ruling by the US Supreme Court made it optional for states. As of March 2019, fourteen states had not expanded their Medicaid programs. This has led to a patchwork situation of coverage. In some states, health care insurance is affordable and offers good coverage, in others, premiums are high, meaning some families would rather forgo the insurance. Before the individual mandate was repealed, this led to financial penalties.

However, given the cost of insurance premiums in these states, those who chose to not be insured ended up paying less in penalties than they might have done so with higher premiums and out-of-pocket costs. In addition, during the first years of the law, younger, healthier individuals didn't exactly flock to the website in droves to sign up for coverage. It was these younger, healthier people who were required to make the bill work. They either opted not to buy the insurance (or paid the penalty, instead) or were able to obtain the necessary insurance they needed through their employers or parents.

On the positive side, the ACA outlined ten essential benefits that private insurance companies were required to cover, under the law (What Marketplace Health Insurance Plans Cover 2016):

- ambulatory patient services
- emergency services
- hospitalization, such as surgery and overnight stays
- pregnancy, maternity, and newborn care
- mental health and substance abuse services
- prescription drugs
- rehabilitative services and devices
- laboratory services
- preventative and wellness services and chronic disease management
- pediatric services, including oral and vision care (however, adult dental and vision coverage aren't considered essential benefits).

In addition, plans also need to cover birth control and breastfeeding.

By 2016, nearly twenty million formerly uninsured Americans had acquired health care coverage through the new health care exchanges or Medicaid expansion (in participating states). Furthermore, the rate of increase in premiums for employer-based health insurance was lower than it had been during the decade before ACA implementation. Research and studies found that in some cases, access to care has increased, as has improvements in self-assessed health.

Still, there is no doubt that the ACA was, and continues to be, a controversial piece of legislation. For one thing, the legislative vote was along party lines (Dorn 2017). Also, much like the Clinton's Health Security Act, the nine-hundred-page ACA was poorly understood by the American public, which didn't receive immediate, tangible benefits from it. As a result, many people developed unfavorable views of the plan, which were exacerbated by the fact that, in the early days, Healthcare.gov, the ACA website, suffered many crashes and bugs, which took a while to fix. Furthermore, Obama's promise that those who liked their insurance could keep it proved to be untrue. Never mind that in many cases, the insurance in question was poor insurance; people were used to it and wanted the option to keep it. Because of these scenarios, the ACA continues, in many cases, to be unfavorably viewed today.

However, one major move forward through the ACA was the preexisting clause. During much of the twentieth century, insurance companies began denying insurance to those with preexisting conditions, including asthma, heart attacks, strokes, and AIDS. The exact point when preexisting conditions became an issue was likely when for-profit insurance companies popped up, but let's remember that in the 1920s, Blue Cross charged the same amount for insurance, regardless of age, sex, or preexisting conditions. As the cost of health care increased, so did the number of people being denied coverage.

Before the ACA passed, it was estimated that one in seven Americans were denied health insurance because of a preexisting condition. Adding insult to injury was that the list of conditions was extensive and many times elusive, depending on what the insurance company wanted to say. The ACA did eliminate the preexisting condition mandate that seemed to be a staple of many insurance companies.

This focus on elimination of preexisting conditions also impacted maternal and prenatal care; previous to the ACA, such care was more restrictive in private insurance policies. Women had to pay an additional fee for maternity coverage for at least twelve months prior to any kind of prenatal care being covered, or else the pregnancy was considered a preexisting condition, and prenatal services were not covered in the policy. As such, while the ACA did have its failings, it was a beginning in the attempt to jump-start health care reform.

◆ Trump and the Republicans: Failure to Overturn

From the moment of the ACA's passage, Republicans in Congress continued to condemn the law, voting more than fifty times in the House of Representatives to repeal or amend it (Levy 2019). It's not clear why the Republicans were so against the law, given that it was actually based on the so-called "Romneycare" of Massachusetts, passed under the leadership of very Republican Governor Mitt Romney. Fears abounded that costs passed on to businesses would end up shrinking the labor pool (despite that fear, this really hasn't happened). But the point was, the Republicans seemed determined to pull apart the bill.

The Republican-controlled Congress's efforts to repeal were largely showboating; the proposals had little or no chance of becoming law, not with President Obama still in office (Hirsch et al. 2017). In point of fact, the ACA had passed without Republican support in either the House or the Senate, and the next several years consisted of Republican-led rallies and legislative efforts with the goal of repealing the ACA. Some of these rallies also included members of the public who had horror stories about how the legislation led to higher premiums and higher medical costs; in some cases, people lost their insurance because it didn't comply with ACA regulations. The issue, however, was that many of the stories simply weren't true, with some of those victims not even checking into the health care exchanges to find out what the legislation was about. Still, Hirsch et al. (2017) said, "Given the rhetoric of the 2016 campaign the eventual election of Donald Trump, Republicans seemed poised to capitalized on this long-standing position" (p. 599).

Donald Trump was elected president in 2016; during his campaign, he promised to replace Obamacare with a plan that would provide all Americans with better coverage and lower premiums. However, House Republicans struggled with coming up with a new bill, as issues under consideration (elimination of the individual mandate, cuts in Medicaid funding, and reduction in advanced tax credits to offset insurance premiums) would cause several million Americans to lose their health insurance.

Divisions in Congress prompted President Trump to sign an executive order in October 2017, permitting the sale of less-expensive health insurance policies with fewer benefits than those required under the law. And the Tax Cuts and Jobs Bill of 2017 effectively repealed the individual mandate by reducing the penalty for not carrying health insurance. This led to a December 2018 ruling by a US district court in Texas, declaring the entire ACA unconstitutional, on the grounds that the individual mandate was unconstitutional, as it could not be enforced as a tax.

During the very contentious campaign season leading up to the 2016 presidential election, Trump proposed to repeal the ACA and replace it with "Healthcare Reform to Make America Great Again"

(Saltzman and Eibner 2016). The focus ranged from allowing individuals to deduct the full amount of premiums for individual health plans from their federal tax returns to allowing insurers to sell insurance across state lines. Yet once Trump won elected office and had a Republican-controlled Congress, he failed to repeal Obamacare several times. What follows are a handful of the more well-known efforts taken in efforts to repeal the ACA since Trump took office:

◆ Part 1: The American Health Care Act

By the time Trump was sworn into office, the Republic Party had full power, enjoying control of the executive branch and both houses of Congress. The Republican Party, which had long blasted the problems they saw with the ACA's deficiencies, now had the means to fix it. Using a budget reconciliation process that had been used to pass major pieces of legislation (such as the above-mentioned COBRA in 1985), in mid-January 2017, Congress voted to allow this process to remove large elements of the ACA and move forward with revising the act (Hirsch et al. 2017).

In early March 2017, a draft of the American Health Care Act (AHCA) was released in the House and almost immediately garnered harsh criticism from many sides, including Democrats, conservative Republicans, patient advocacy groups, the American Medical Association, and the American Hospital Association. Far-right conservatives, including the House Freedom Caucus, sneeringly called the proposed act "Obamacare Lite," while many moderates and liberals claimed it would jeopardize insurance coverage for millions of Americans.

One of the issues of concerns involved capping Medicaid support after 2020. Basically, the ACHA mandated that states accepting Medicaid expansion would continue receiving federal funds for beneficiaries joining Medicaid until 2020. After that time, states wouldn't be permitted to accept new expansion enrollees, which would increase the numbers of the uninsured. Furthermore, some states still hadn't accepted expanded Medicaid under the ACA. For those states, the AHCA would have provided "safety-net funding" allowing the states to increase payments to Medicaid providers from 2018 to 2022.

Then there was the individual mandate; the ACHA indicated, unequivocally, that it would be repealed. However, it wouldn't have repealed current protections for people with preexisting conditions, instead, issuing a so-called "continuous coverage" requirement that permitted insurers to impose a penalty on individuals who allowed their health care coverage to lapse.

The ACHA also would have gotten rid of the various insurance subsidies offered through the Affordable Care Act, for those earning a lower income. Instead, the new law would have replaced the subsidies with age-based credits; basically, regardless of premiums, the bill would have provided insurance purchasers with a refundable tax credit that increased with age. The credits could have been used for insurance plans that weren't involved with the state exchanges, and credits would be reduced and eliminated, based on progressively higher income. Finally, the ACHA would have encouraged the use of health care saving accounts (HSAs), which are used to pay for out-of-pocket health care expenses.

While the ACHA also repealed the ACA's requirement that

insurers classify their plans as gold, silver, or bronze (depending on the share of health costs covered by the plan), it once again did not impact the preexisting condition provision, nor would it have prohibited children from staying on their parents' health insurance policies until age twenty-six. The Congressional Budget Office (CBO) released a statement in mid-March 2017, indicating that the ACHA would reduce the federal deficit by $337 billion over a ten-year period (that amount diminished to $186 billion, after the bill was modified during House debate).

However, the Republican effort was stymied by the above-mentioned House Freedom Caucus, which disliked the Affordable Care Act from the get-go. The caucus, consisting of ultra-conservative Republicans who didn't want any form of government intervention in health care, wasn't happy with the American Health Care Act. Their complaints ranged from wanting fewer insurance requirements to repealing essential benefits to Title 1 of the ACA, which promised "quality, affordable healthcare for all Americans." Title 1, incidentally, was the foundation of the ACA, and it's somewhat confusing why the caucus wanted to do away with that aspect of the plan.

The Trump administration, along with House Majority Leader Paul Ryan, attempted to make changes to the bill that would bring in support from the Freedom Caucus and other groups. Once such idea involved repeal of the ten essential benefits, but this risked alienating the more moderate Republicans. The essential benefits were yet another cornerstone of Obamacare, and Republicans knew they risked constituents' ire if they voted against it.

Speaking of constituents, Republicans were gradually under fire from the people who sent them to Washington DC in the first place, due to fears that the ACHA would lead to a rise in uninsured individuals (Hirsch et al. 2017). Ryan withdrew the bill in late March, due to a lack of House Republican support. Digging more deeply, several reasons stand out as to this potential legislation's demise, including the inability to compromise with congressional Democrats, who were reluctant to replace and repeal the ACA, which was the signature legislation of the most recent Democratic president. Many agreed that the law had a variety of challenges; however, they believed it made better sense to modify and improve the existing law, rather than replacing it with something else.

There also was an inability to craft the legislation with language that could appeal to both parties. Republicans needed to use the reconciliation process to propose the bill (Hirsch et al. 2017). Without that language, the Democrats had every reason to use a filibuster tool to prevent a vote from taking place. Campaign promises made by Trump were opposite of the reality of the Republican-controlled Congress. When Trump was campaigning for president, he made several promises regarding health care and how he would fix the ACA, once he was elected to office. One of his promises was that he would provide insurance to everyone; he also said there would be no cuts to Medicare, Medicaid, and Social Security, which were contrary to many Republicans' views. ACHA didn't exactly live up to Trump's campaign promises. This, in turn, generated anger among constituents, who had been promised one thing but given another.

To summarize, the ACHA died because congressional Republicans couldn't think of a way to pass it. Appealing to the more conservative House Freedom Caucus alienated more moderate

Republicans, and vice versa. The fractured Republican Party, along with the fact that the public was actually becoming more used to working within the parameters of the Affordable Care Act, doomed the bill to failure.

◆ Part 2: Better Care Reconciliation Act

During the summer of 2017, the ACHA rose like a phoenix from the ashes. This time, the Republican-controlled Senate took the lead on "repeal-and-replace" legislation. Dubbed the Better Care Reconciliations Act (BCRA) of 2017, the bill included two tax provisions from the ACA and additional factors that would help pay for low-income insurance premiums (Morgan and Nicholson 2017). Once the procedural challenges were met, the Senate planned to vote on the original ACHA. The new, revised ACHA also included proposals to offset costs, which included premium stabilization, a Better Care Reconciliation Implementation Fund, and an addition of catastrophic plans. The legislation was geared toward repealing the ACA's spending on insurance coverage, as well as getting rid of taxes on the wealthy and health care industries. However, the CBO, when analyzing the new legislation, pointed out that that it also would have meant thirty-two million fewer Americans with health care insurance by 2027, without some kind of replacement (Scott 2017).

The BCRA was yet another repeal-and-replace, but it failed to pass in late July, as nine Republicans opposed it. At the same time, the Obamacare Repeal Reconciliation Act, considered a "cleaner" bill by some Republicans, also failed, with seven Republicans and all Democrats voting to block it. As a note, part of the issue here involved efforts by Sen. Ted Cruz (R-Texas) to add a proposal allowing insurers to sell less-expensive, bare-bones plans with those that complied with stricter requirements from the ACA. Furthermore, Sen. Rob Portman (R-Ohio), added another proposal to the plan: to move low-income people off Medicaid and onto private insurance.

However, the CBO didn't score either the Cruz or Portman proposals, and the proposals were voted down. Other bills came forward, including a so-called "skinny repeal," that focused on a narrower proposal. However, the Senate was unable to come to an agreement on any of these bills.

◆ Part 3: Graham-Cassidy Bill

In September 2017, in an attempt to try yet again to focus on getting rid of Obamacare, Bill Cassidy (R-Louisiana), Lindsey O. Graham (R-South Carolina), Dean Heller (R-Nevada), and Ron Johnson (R-Wisconsin) introduced yet another repeal-and-replace effort, this one known as the Graham-Cassidy Bill (Soffen 2017). Rather than funding Medicaid and subsidies directly, Graham-Cassidy noted that money would be put into a block grant to states which would, in turn, be used to develop any health care system it wanted. The proposal also allowed states to opt out of many ACA regulations. While Graham claimed that those liking their ACA insurance could keep it, the cutting of both Medicaid expansion and subsidy funding ensured that costs would increase. And as with other ACA repeal-and-replacement bills, the individual mandate would be eliminated. Furthermore, insurance companies would be able to

charge older customers up to five times as much as younger customers (versus the ACA, which mandated that older customers would be
charged only as much as three times as younger consumers).

However, like other attempts to repeal and replace Obamacare,
the bill didn't pass; Senate Majority Leader Mitch McConnell, in
fact, skewered it, once again, fearing that not enough votes were in
place to pass it. The bill ran into the same fate that had killed the
other bills, namely, that many Republicans were wary of changing
the US health care system in such a haphazard process. Other issues
not to their liking included proposed deep cuts to Medicaid, as well
as roll-back protections for individuals with preexisting conditions.

Furthermore, and adding problems to Graham-Lindsay, were
last-minute changes to the bill, which made senators wary about
voting on it. They didn't have much time to thoroughly study it (or,
at the very least, their aides didn't have the time to do so). Much
like the other attempts to repeal Obamacare, it seemed as though
Graham-Lindsay was somewhat of a slap-dash affair, and effort to
get something through, so they could honor campaign pledges to
constituents about getting rid of Obamacare.

The above represents the most well-known efforts the
Republicans attempted to repeal Obamacare. Throughout 2017,
other legislation and efforts were tried, but they met the similar fate
of the above three pieces of legislation. So why did the Republicans
fail so spectacularly in their efforts to repeal and replace a bill that
was so loathed by much of the party?

One major reason was the Republican Party itself. Quite simply,
various party factions couldn't agree on a reasonable substitute for
the ACA, and that disagreement ended up stimming any reasonable

reform. President Obama, on the other hand, was able to bridge the split between Democratic Party purists and centrists to push the ACA through, even as the repeal-and-replace efforts failed among Republicans (Bendavid 2017). For another thing, back in 2009–2010, when the ACA was making its tortuous way through chambers of government and town hall meetings, Democrats were able to bring the health industry and medical associations on board to support the bill. They did so by promising new markets and financial help when it came to implementing the ACA. In addition, the AMA didn't perceive that the ACA would end up cutting physician wages, while private insurance companies were informed that they would still be able to earn profits.

However, those same groups largely were against the GOP bills, especially with their focus on entitlement cutbacks and potential cuts in profits and physician salaries. Also bringing up a sour note was Trump's proposed cuts to the Medicaid program, which didn't sit right with many Republican governors. Finally, the Democrats fully expected to win the 2008 presidential election, which they did. As such, the party (and the Democrat-controlled Congress) was able to successfully push health care as a top priority. The party had a full-fledged proposal, and a plan on how to pass it through the political process, at the ready.

Fast-forwarding eight years, however, many Republicans didn't expect Trump to be elected president and, as such, didn't have a full health proposal ready. Noted Naftali Bendavid, "Health care was Mr. Obama's clear priority for his first term, and Democrats spent more than a year on it, while Republican leaders sought to move quickly on health care to pave the way for a tax overhaul."

One might wonder why, if the Republicans had spent seven years since the passage of the ACA bemoaning its existence and threatening to push it back through highly publicized showboating efforts, they didn't have an actual plan ready to put into place when the time came. That particular issue is beyond the scope of this book. However, the struggle to get the ACA passed, as well as the many, many attempts lawmakers have attempted to debunk or roll it back, speaks to the highly politicized arena in which health care reform exists. As such, simply suggesting that health care be reformed isn't enough. If a health care reform proposal is to succeed, it would require inputs from myriad stakeholders, all with varying different agendas, thoughts, and beliefs. As the repeal-and-replace aspect of the ACA proved, even those within the same party often can't agree on a logical solution.

Another wrinkle concerning health care, in general, and the Affordable Care Act, in particular, is the general public's belief about it. A better word might be "confusion." In some cases, the people who sneered at Obamacare and supported the Republicans' efforts to overturn it were the same people who actually benefitted from the Affordable Care Act. This is because many Americans didn't understand that Obamacare and the ACA were one and the same. According to a Morning Consult poll, 35 percent said they either thought Obamacare and the ACA were different policies or didn't know if they were the same or different (Dropp and Nyhan 2017). This confusion was especially pronounced among people eighteen to twenty years old and those who earned less than fifty thousand dollars: "two groups that could significantly be affected by repeal" (Dropp and Nyhan 2017).

Furthermore, when respondents were asked what would happen if Obamacare were repealed, approximately 45 percent didn't know that the ACA would be repealed. Perhaps unsurprisingly, knowledge of policy consequences of repeal without replacement differed sharply along party/partisan lines. Noted Morning Consult's Kyle Dropp, "This confusion may affect the public debate over health care policy. If many people think repealing Obamacare would not affect the popular provisions of the A.C.A., they might not understand the potential consequences of the proposals being considered in Washington" (2019).

Meanwhile, President Trump continues chipping away at the ACA, with the most recent activity coming from the Department of Justice, which gave its full backing to a legal repeal of the act (Tozzi and Wasson 2019). The administration has also succeeded in weakening some of the key planks of the law, including using the Tax Cuts and Jobs Act of 2017 to eliminate the ACA's individual mandate: the financial penalty in place for failing to buy health insurance. The mandate, which focused on insuring every man, woman, and child in the United States, was a signature piece of the bill. However, there have been issues concerning the constitutionality of forcing everyone to buy insurance, when they might not want to; the argument about this involves the rights of individuals.

Additionally, while President Obama and the federal government spent days and weeks before the deadline encouraging people to enroll in health care plans for the next year, Trump and his federal government haven't done much in the way of outreach. In fact, Trump narrowed the enrollment period, making it more difficult for people to enroll in insurance. Some states have opted out of running local ACA exchanges, meaning the enrollment processes are up to the federal government. This also means a patchwork of enrollment; while California residents, for example, can enroll in health care through January 15, Texas, which does not have state-run exchanges, is following the federal enrollment deadline of December 15.

In addition, federal spending to promote ACA enrollment has been cut from $163 million to $20 million; this means less advertising encouraging individuals to enroll, as well as grants provided to nongovernmental groups to assist people in enrollments. Still, the American people are not willing to buy into the political argument of getting rid of Obamacare.

We've gone into a great deal of detail over both the passage of the ACA and its attempted repeal to demonstrate the difficulty in developing and passing any kind of meaningful health care reform. The flurry of bills and counter bills during 2017 proved how difficult it was for the Republicans (who controlled the executive and legislative branches) to get their agendas and legislation through.

As we continually mention, part of the problem involved fissures in the Republican Party; specifically, the House Freedom Caucus couldn't see eye-to-eye with more moderate Republicans. The end result was that by early 2018, Republican leadership wasn't even interested in trying yet another repeal-and-replace effort, for fear that there wouldn't be enough votes to pass it. The issue has gotten even more troublesome for Republicans now, especially as the Democrats took back the House majority during the 2018 midterm elections.

Still, steps have been taken to try to chip away at the bill, one of which was the above-referenced lawsuit against the law (once again) being unconstitutional. Basically, as flawed as Obamacare is, people are used to it now. And as with other issues about the health care system that people are used to, once these issues are in place, they are difficult to change. The discussion above focuses on the problems in passing any kind of health care reform. The question at this point isn't whether universal coverage or a single-payer system will work. Rather, it focuses on whether legislation can be passed by Congress, agreed to by the president, and then passed into meaningful law. To get to that point, many special-interest groups need to be appeased, making reform of the health care system massively difficult. Obamacare ran into a great deal of criticism. So did Medicare and Medicaid and Social Security. These days, however, these programs are accepted as part of the fabric of society. So, to an extent, is the ACA. Basically, once they make it to the mainstream and are out there for a while, the American people become used to it.

Political obstacles have remained when it comes to repairing/ repealing the ACA (Dorn 2017). Dorn, for one, pointed out that "it took progressives decades to pass a comprehensive health reform bill.... Opponents of the ACA have been trying to do something even more difficult: Replacing an established entitlement program that, now, under threat, is more popular than ever" (p. 1,466).

CHAPTER FOUR: WHERE WE ARE NOW

◆ The ACA Today

EVEN AS BICKERING CONTINUES IN WASHINGTON DC over health care reform (and the Democratic Party is attempting to come up with solutions to the problem in hopes of winning the 2020 presidency), the question is whether the ACA has been effective in providing more coverage and reducing costs. The answer is, it depends.

There is no doubt that Obamacare has meant more than twenty million Americans gained health coverage (Sanger-Katz 2017). It has reduced inequality, providing lower-income Americans with the opportunity to secure health care coverage at more reasonable rates. The law has also made health insurance more comprehensive; for example, health plans are required to cover maternity care and treatment for drug addiction. Finally, it has lowered the federal deficit.

Obamacare has not, however, achieved uniform affordability; as mentioned throughout this book, health care in the United State remains the most expensive in the world. Furthermore, coverage is out of the financial reach of many US citizens. Basically, health insurance remains very expensive. While those who are fortunate enough to have health insurance as part of their benefit package don't seem to be feeling the pinch, those who are earning too much to be above the poverty line continue to struggle to pay health plan premiums and face deductibles that are higher than those seen in a typical employer health plan. The families that must work two and three part-time jobs in an effort to make ends meet, or who are working for employers that don't offer health insurance as a benefit, are the ones that continue to suffer, even with the Affordable Care Act in place.

In many cases, the ACA did not cover individuals with incomes over 400 percent of the federal poverty level (less than $100,000 a year for a household of four) (Hirsch et al. 2017). This group of people doesn't qualify for Medicaid or for federal subsidies to purchase insurance on the ACA-created health exchange. As a result, these families have been forced to purchase high-cost, unsubsidized insurance.

Furthermore, the health care system remains complex and confusing. Selecting the right health plan is frustrating or impossible for many Americans, with terms such as "out-of-pocket maximum" or "in-network provider" not making things much easier. Added Sanger-Katz, "After picking their insurance, patients can still struggle to use it, and get stuck with surprise bills or long negotiations with their insurance companies" (2017). Even after paying premiums and co-pays, in other words, patients can be—and often are—still on the hook for full payment, at least until they meet their deductibles. And despite the ACA's positive intentions, the legislation's very complex regulatory framework has been blamed for increasing out-of-pocket costs and deductibles for many patients, both on exchanges and on employer-based health care plans.

For one thing, the ten essential benefits, while important, have meant added services and costs, which insurance companies have been all too happy to pass along to customers and employers. These added services have also ended up contributing to affordability challenges for individuals who have employer-based insurance. Another aspect to consider is that while employer-based insurance is non-taxable, individuals working for those employers are required to purchase their portion of the insurance with their post-tax dollars, which provides additional problems.

In short, the ACA involves "a patchwork-style reform that built on the existing health care system" (Dorn 2017, p. 1,465). The difficulty here is that the existing system was already a mess before Obamacare came along. Furthermore, the ACA's problems rest within the individual insurance market. In some instances (and many states), insurance beneficiaries have been subject to high deductibles or a limited choice of physicians, reflecting a policy failure. Additionally, similar to the early days of ACA implementation, the individual mandate and premium subsidies haven't been effective in getting younger, healthier individuals to sign up for coverage. The result is that insurance risk pools are weighed toward older, sicker, and more costly members who can no longer be denied coverage or charged premiums in line with risk. This explains why insurance companies have been so willing to charge more for premiums.

Adding to the problem has been political opposition in some states when it comes to health care exchanges and a refusal to fund risk corridors that would offset losses. Finally, insurance companies, themselves, aren't competent when it comes to managing actuarial risk, especially for low-income people in nongroup, state-based markets. Some markets are unattractive to many insurers, prompting them to leave those markets. The few insurance companies that remain can raise premiums because there is, in a sense, no competition to do otherwise. As such, when it comes to this particular policy goal, the ACA has been a dismal failure.

To summarize, yes, the Affordable Care Act has boosted insurance coverage for many who need it. On the other hand, it is leading to higher premiums as well as higher out-of-pocket costs. Getting a handle on health care involves more than mandating that everyone has insurance. Rather, it needs to attack one of the main issues of US health care: unsustainable high costs.

◆ High Costs, Intertwined with Profits

One of the central problems with a market-driven health care system (which the United States supposedly has) is that there are fewer providers, hospitals, and health care facilities than there is demand. Economics 101 indicates that when supply of a service doesn't increase with the demand for that service, the price of that service will increase. This is what is happening with health care in the United States. Because of increased demand, yet not an increase in supply, prices are skyrocketing. The end result here is that rather than improving the product (health care) or improving the logistic system (delivery of health care), the free market enterprise of health care has translated into a decline in actual health care conditions (because they can) and an increase in cost. This has translated into poor health care in many urban centers and also created a system that makes illness prevention cost-prohibitive to the underinsured or uninsured.

It's less expensive for an insurance company to cover a particular medicine to prevent a heart attack than having patients have a heart attack and end up in the hospital because they couldn't afford the medicine the insurance company refused to cover. This type of thing is counterintuitive, yet it goes on all the time. Bartlett and Steele (2004) maintain that the government has turned the issue over to the private organizations and asked them to sort out the profit-driven process through which health care has developed.

As health care organizations and hospitals nationwide become moneymaking devices, the number of people served and the level of care have declined. In these corporate monstrosities, health care is both a service and a commodity, and so health care organizations have rejected a consumer focus and focused on profit. Rather than creating a level of competitiveness, as suggested in the Reagan administration's call for a focus on market-driven health care, the health care system is driven by such a great profit motive that it becomes easy to reject a compassionate response to the care needs of the many and seek out ways of providing care for those who can pay the most for it. This does little, if anything, to improve health outcomes for the population as a whole.

Physicians for a National Healthcare Plan (PNHP) point out that while the ACA has good intentions and reduced co-payments and deductibles for families that have incomes 100–250 percent of the poverty line, "the financial burden on the middle class will remain high" (PNHP 2016). The organization also pointed out that bronze plans purchased through exchanges have covered, on average, only 60 percent of enrollees' expenses, leaving families to bear out-of-pocket costs of up to $13,200 annually for covered services, not including premiums (PNHP 2016). As mentioned earlier, premiums and out-of-pocket costs have been so high that some families are preferring to go without insurance. This has been worsened in some states that have refused to expand Medicaid, while imposing increased out-of-pocket costs on Medicaid recipients (PNHP 2016). Even worse, the PHNP noted that expanded coverage under the ACA will likely increase bureaucracy, funneling an estimated $895 billion in new federal subsidies (and billions more in family-paid premiums) to private insurers, "reinforcing their grip on care, and wasting billions on their overhead."

Finally, there is the issue of Medicaid expansion coverage under the ACA, mentioned earlier. Many states have opted to expand Medicaid coverage under the act, while others have not. The result is that in one state offering expanded coverage, a family can get away with paying lower premiums for health care coverage (not to mention lower out-of-cost deductibles and co-pays), whereas in another state, in which the coverage hasn't expanded, that same family is subject to extraordinarily high premiums, as well as escalating out-of-pocket costs and co-payments.

The website howmuch.net recently compared annual insurance deductibles through an ACA silver plan. Florida came in at the highest, with $6,913 a year, whereas Pennsylvania's annual deductible was $1,733 (How Much 2018). Noted the website, "While the health insurance debate takes place at the national level, health insurance rates actually vary between states." Again, this goes back to the very patchwork nature of health care, in general, not to mention the Affordable Care Act. What about solutions that the ACA provided to rein in the higher costs? These solutions, Accountable Care Organizations (ACOs) and Value-Based Payment (VBO)/Pay for Performance systems, were put into place as cost-effective measures. Following are explanations of these plans and an assessment of their effectiveness.

◆ Accountable Care Organizations

ACOs are Medicare programs and are one way in which the ACA has sought to reduce health care costs. The ACO model encourages health care providers, hospitals, and others to form networks that help better coordinate patient care (Gold 2015). The idea here is that as networks deliver care more efficiently, they can become eligible for bonuses. This is because the networks share financial and medical responsibility for coordinated care, which in theory should limit unnecessary duplication of effort and spending. For instance, instead of many specialists running many blood tests on a single patient, the ACO means one blood draw, with the many specialists making their analysis from that draw. Under this system, the healthier they keep their patients, the more providers can earn.

The working theory behind the ACO is the very fragmented health care system of the United States. Patients obtain their health care separately, from different providers, meaning different bills. A visit to the emergency room is a good case in point. The patient will likely receive multiple bills from such a visit, such as the emergency room bill and a bill from a doctor. If a specialist is called in, that is another bill. And if that visit requires surgery, this opens up a whole host of other bills from the surgeon, the anesthesiologist, and anyone else involved with the procedure. ACOs, however, are supposed to reduce this type of issue.

While ACOs don't do away with fee-for-service programs, they do create an incentive to offer bonuses when providers keep costs down. ACOs are required to maintain benchmarks and provide extensive reporting of quality indicators, with some payments withheld unless specific quality targets are met (PNHP 2016; see also Nash 2018). With more ACOs cropping up in the private sector as well as within Medicare practices, the question has been whether they've been effective. The evidence, so far, shows that the Medicare Shared Savings Program—the largest value-based payment model in the country—has ACOs that have improved quality and saved money for the Medicare program. Even better news, it seems, is that "spillover effects from these ACOs appear to be changing care delivery ... [while] lowering cost growth in local healthcare markets."

Still, there have been concerns among health care economists that formation of ACOs could lead to more hospital mergers and consolidations (in other words, more monopolization of health care). Hospitals, in an effort to become integrated systems, are purchasing independent physician practices, meaning fewer independent hospitals and doctors are available to care for patients. Greater market share means the health systems have more leverage in insurer negotiations, which can, in the end, drive up health costs, while limiting patient choice.

Additionally, the disagreement as to actual effectiveness is centered on the degree of cost savings that the Medicare Shared Savings

Program (MSSP) ACOs have achieved. While the Center for Medicare & Medicaid indicated that MSSP ACOs generated $954 million in savings, independent researchers suspect this actually underestimates the actual ACOs money savings, claiming the savings are actually $1.8 billion. This does seem to be good news on the surface, but Kip Sullivan (2018) didn't buy any of it. He noted that in a report from the Centers for Medicare and Medicaid Services on its Medicare ACO programs, data from 2016 showed that the programs were breaking even, "and that's only if you don't count the costs to the ACOs of doing whatever it is ACOs do," Sullivan commented. The report focused on so-called "pioneer" ACOs, of which several had dropped out of the program, over time. Furthermore, a pilot program with ACO Physician Group Practice noted that the ACO saved Medicare 0.3 percent of the claims amounts, while performance payments were 1.5 percent of the claims amounts.

On the one hand, ACOs do seem to be saving some money, yet on the other hand, research seems to indicate that other costs are not being considered when it comes to reports from these programs. Sullivan, once again, indicated that the costs of setting up ACOs to begin with can be quite high, and those costs aren't necessarily reflected in the entire reporting amount. As such, while the theory behind such organizations is a nice one, the reality seems to be something different.

◆ Value-Based Payment

The other aspect of the Affordable Care Act is the concept of value-based payment, sometimes known as value-based health care. Value-based payment is a health care delivery model in which health care providers are paid based on patient health outcomes (What Is Value-Based Healthcare 2017). Providers are rewarded when they help patients improve health, reduce the impact and incidence of chronic diseases, and live healthier lives (What Is Value-Based Healthcare 2017). Rather than a fee-for-service or capitated approach to medicine and health care delivery, VBP providers are paid based on the amount of health care services they deliver, with the value derived from measuring health outcomes against the costs of delivering those outcomes.

The purported benefit of value-based health care is that patients spend less money to achieve better health (as the focus involves avoiding chronic disease in the first place); providers can achieve greater efficiencies and higher patient satisfaction; and payers are better able to control costs and reduce risks, by spreading that risk across a larger patient population. A healthier patient population leads to fewer claims, meaning less drain on payers' premium pools and investments, and fewer administrative costs affiliated with operations. Meanwhile, suppliers align prices with patient outcomes, meaning reduced costs.

The idea behind value-based payment is a good one; however, the PNHP pointed out that "it rests on dubious assumptions about measurement and motivation." Basically, attempting to understand genetic, social, and behavioral factors that influence health can be difficult, and no "foreseeable risk-adjustment algorithm reliably accounts for the many patient factors that are beyond a clinicians' control," the PNHP pointed out (2016). This is probably correct; for example, a physician who requires a patient to attempt a smoking cessation clinic can't guarantee that the patient will be weaned off cigarettes forever, despite that doctor's best efforts and intentions. Unless the patient wants to quit smoking, no amount of nicotine gum, doctor nagging, patches, or classes will help.

ACOs and VBPs aren't the only disappointments coming from the ACA. One main issue is that the coverage gains under the law haven't come from the private plans offered in the marketplaces (Hacker 2018). Rather, those gains have come from Medicaid, the government program that was expanded under the law (Hacker 2018). Medicaid enrollment exceeded expectations, meaning the CBO's overall projections for increased coverage have panned out, despite disappointing individual marketplace numbers. The Medicaid program is now larger than Medicare, consisting of almost seventy-five million enrollees, including those covered by the Children's Health Insurance Program (CHIP).

But once again, this only takes into account the states that accepted Medicaid expansion. Nineteen (Republican-controlled) states continue to refuse to expand Medicaid, and other conservative states continue working to actively undermine enrollment in individual marketplaces. I already mentioned that while President Obama was in office, congressional Republicans voted more than fifty times to kill the ACA. The Republicans also sued the president to stop subsidy payments (Hacker 2018). In addition, Republicans have failed to appropriate funds to boost marketplace enrollment and, overall, turned their consistent warnings about the ACA's failures into a self-fulfilling prophecy. Republicans also continue dragging their feet on reauthorizing CHIP, which once had overall strong bipartisan support.

CHAPTER FIVE: THE US HEALTH CARE SYSTEM TODAY

WE'VE SPENT A LOT OF TIME REVIEWING THE HISTORY OF health care and health care reform in the United States, as well as focusing on the Affordable Care Act. However, before we can study specific health care reforms, we need to understand the system, itself. While the current cry of "Medicare for All" has a nice ring to it, in truth, many challenges stand in the way of achieving that goal. The main challenge is the makeup of the health care system, itself.

◆ Health Care Delivery

In explaining problems with health care delivery in America, Porter and Lee (2013) point to a common ailment, that of back pain. One patient suffering from an aching back might visit her primary care physician. Another (depending on insurance) might opt to go straight to the orthopedist. A third might consider a chiropractor or even a neurologist. Depending on that visit, the patients might be referred to a specialist. Or perhaps X-rays or an MRI might be called for. In some cases, physical therapy or surgery might be prescribed. These various patchwork options come into play for a patient with a basic backache, not a life-threatening illness. But in the US health care system, this simple problem ends up generating encounters with different health care providers, all separate from one another, with no one entity coordinating the entire care. As such, "duplication of effort, delays and inefficiency is almost inevitable," Porter and Lee note.

Now, think about this duplication of effort when it comes to serious illnesses, such as pancreatic cancer, and the number of providers, from the oncologists, to the nurse practitioners, to the pharmacists, to the radiologists involved in such treatment. This, of course, leads to separate billings from each provider, meaning the patient receives a plethora of paperwork for each service, thus adding to the administrative costs. While the managed care concept sought to reduce this issue by using the primary care physician as a gatekeeper for additional services, this wasn't effective either; many times, the decisions made at the primary care level weren't the correct ones because they weren't the most profitable ones. The ACOs, discussed above, are attempting to coordinate care. However, at this time, it's too soon to determine their success.

Porter and Lee also pointed out that the fragmentation of health care delivery means there are few, if any, metrics when it comes to patient outcomes. A lack of measurement of these outcomes means uncertainty when it comes to best evidence-based practices. Returning to our sore-backed patient, it could mean uncertainty as to how long the process might take to mitigate the pain. The end result is confusion over what specific care might cost and the idea that the value of the care rarely, if ever, improves.

◆ Employer-Sponsored Health Care

Many US citizens receive their health insurance through their employers. As mentioned above, the employer-sponsored plans took off during World War II; with wages frozen due to government decree, businesses relied on benefits, such as paid health insurance, to compete for talent and labor (Carroll 2017). In 1943, the IRS decided that employer-based health insurance should be exempt from taxation, meaning it became easier to obtain health insurance through a job rather than through other means.

Yet, more than seventy years after World War II ended, the employer-sponsored insurance from the 1940s doesn't exist, any more than health care from that period exists. Those with employer-sponsored health care insurance face the following issues:

Job lock. Because people become dependent on their employment for health insurance, they are reluctant to leave their jobs, even if finding a better job might better their lives. Many are afraid that the market exchange coverage might not be as good as what they have, and more often than not, they are right. Furthermore, fears of the repeal of the Affordable Care Act adds to concerns they might not find affordable insurance at all.

An expensive system. The single-largest tax expenditure in the United States is for employer-based health insurance, which is even more expensive than the mortgage interest deduction. In 2017, the exclusion cost the federal government approximately $260 billion in lost income and payroll taxes, significantly more than the annual cost of the Affordable Care Act.

A regressive system. The tax break for employer-sponsored health insurance is worth more to people who earn more than to those who earn little. The current system also means employers are spending more on health insurance, meaning less money is available to increase wages. Many economists believe that employer-sponsored health insurance is negatively impacting Americans' paychecks.

The system punishes small businesses. It's one thing for larger corporations when it comes to health insurance affordability. However, small businesses are less able to manage the financial burden of helping to provide health insurance to their employers, and according to the Small Business & Enterprise Council, a good many businesses in America are small businesses. Specifically, firms with fewer than five hundred workers accounted for 99.7 percent of the 5.6 million employer firms in the United States, firms with fewer than a hundred workers accounted for 98.2 percent, and firms with fewer than twenty workers made up 89 percent (Facts & Data on Small Business and Entrepreneurship 2017).

Insurance premiums are a huge overhead cost for all businesses; it represents an even larger cost for smaller businesses. David Steil, a small business owner, noted that while the burden of health insurance continues falling on businesses, not all businesses can manage those high costs. In 2016, only 56 percent of businesses could provide employer-sponsored coverage; even worse was that only 46 percent of small businesses had any kind of budget for employer-sponsored health insurance (Steil 2018). "The responsibility of business owners to provide insurance to their employees is putting a strain on their budgets," Steil commented, adding that such a strain makes it difficult to increase wages or plan for long-term growth. The result is that people have no coverage, or they have coverage that is so expensive, they can't afford to use it. "Our healthcare system is hurting our economy and our country," he remarked.

Lack of expertise to manage the burden. While larger employers have been successfully able to actually run and manage their own insurance plans and health bills, most employers don't have the staff or the expertise to oversee the intricacies of health care markets (Blumenthal 2017). Furthermore, even large employers have little bargaining power with insurance and coverage, as their workforces count for only a small portion of the providers' overall markets.

Employers also don't work together to increase leverage with insurance providers; they are, after all, focused on their own businesses, and in some cases, laws prevent them from collaborating. So employers, in attempts to limit their exposure to health care costs, are shifting more of those costs to their employees. This, in turn, has led to an increase in the number of Americans with employer-sponsored health plans who are underinsured. This group is reporting health care access and medical bill problems at close to the same rates as adults who have lacked overall coverage. David Blumenthal said, "If employer-sponsored health insurance continues to become less and less adequate over time ... the discontent of the middle-class working Americans with the cost of their health care will inevitably increase."

There is already evidence that this is taking place. In 2017, after enrollment for the ACA ended, consumers in many states looked for individual coverage and had limited options (Freeman 2017). The reason? Higher utilization costs led insurers to pull out of various markets because policies were unprofitable. The end result was private insurers in some of states only offered plans with high premiums and higher deductibles. Basically, insurance companies are pushing away consumers, as they continue to work around the Affordable Care Act's challenges to profitability, with the end result being that consumers—especially middle-class consumers—struggling to be able to pay for insurance.

To summarize, the idea of employer-sponsored health insurance, which has been the bedrock of the United States for decades, is crumbling. Rising health care costs and premiums are forcing many businesses to pass costs on to their employees who, in turn, might not be able to afford plans with lower deductibles. Other businesses aren't even bothering, which is forcing employees to find other alternatives or to do without. Much like the current runaway prices of the US health care system, employer-sponsored health insurance isn't a sustainable way to cover people.

◆ Health Care and Poverty

One difficulty with any kind of insurance/health care reform in the United States is that it doesn't address root causes of the problem. One of those problems is poverty: There is a definite link between income and health. This shouldn't come as a surprise, but recent studies and trends have solidified this idea. For one thing, income inequality has increased in recent decades, with health indicators at a plateau (Khullar and Chokshi 2018). Life expectancies also differ by income. One study pointed out that since 2001, life expectancy increased by about 2.5 years for the top 5 percent of the income distribution. Meanwhile, there have been no gains for the bottom 5 percent. Men in the top 1 percent of the income distribution can expect to live fifteen years longer than those in the bottom 1 percent. And for women, the difference is about ten years.

Poor adults in the United States are five times as likely as those with incomes above 400 percent of the federal poverty level to report being in poor or fair health. Low-income Americans report higher rates of physical limitations and heart disease, diabetes, stroke, and other chronic conditions, compared to higher-income Americans. Per Khullar and Chokshi, "For the 6.8 million children living in deep poverty ... there are adverse consequences across the life course related to nutrition, environmental exposures, chronic illness and language development." Furthermore, education, employment, race, ethnicity, and even geography are shown to influence health outcomes. And finally, current health care payment and delivery system reforms are encouraging an emphasis on addressing social health determinants, including income. Let's see how this manifests itself; income influences health, which can be divided into clinical, behavioral, and environmental factors.

Compared to higher-income Americans, low-income people face greater barriers when it comes to accessing medical care. This demographic is less likely to have health insurance, to receive new drugs or technologies, and to have ready access to primary or specialty care. Low-income workers are more likely to be employed by organizations that don't offer health care benefits. Less than one-third of low-income workers obtain health insurance through their employers, compared to nearly 60 percent of higher-income workers.

Even after implementation of the Affordable Care Act, more than twenty-seven million Americans remain uninsured. The majority of these are low-income people; those without health insurance are less likely to have a regular source of medical care and are more likely to forgo care due to cost concerns. Low-income Americans have higher rates of behavioral risk factors, such as smoking, obesity, substance abuse, and low levels of physical activity. Poorer neighborhoods have a higher density of tobacco retailers and have less access to fresh foods, a higher density of fast-food restaurants, and an environment that is not conducive to physical activity. Finally, low-income Americans tend to have daily environmental exposures that create wear and tear on the body through repeated and chronic stressors. These include higher levels of violence, discrimination, and material deprivation, such as lack of housing, heat, water, or electricity.

The relationship between race and income and health continues. Low-income black Americans live shorter lives than high-income black Americans, though affluent blacks die earlier than affluent whites. Other racial and ethnic groups, such as Hispanic Americans and American Indians, have lower incomes, fewer educational opportunities, and shorter life expectancies than whites. Having said that, most Americans with low incomes are white, and low-income white Americans have been impacted in the largest numbers by the opioid epidemic, which is thought to be partly responsible for recent decreases in US live expectancy.

The reason why health care reform has been so difficult to implement boils down to politics and the idea that a one-size-fits-all approach simply isn't effective. Specifically, a multifaceted policy approach is necessary for truly meaningful reform. But wasn't the Affordable Care Act supposed to assist lower-income individuals? Yes, but as mentioned earlier, some of that assistance came in the form of the Medicaid health care exchange, which is a joint program between the federal and state governments. Many states opted to implement Medicare expansion under the ACA; many, however, did not. In these states, Medicaid eligibility under the ACA is limited; the median income limit for parents in these states is just 43 percent of poverty, or an annual income of $8,935 (Garfield, Orgera, and Damico 2019). In nearly all states that did not expand Medicaid coverage, childless adults are not eligible.

Also, because the ACA's intent was to provide coverage to low-income people through Medicaid, the act doesn't provide financial assistance to people below the poverty level for other coverage options. This means that in states that didn't expand Medicaid options, many families and childless adults fall into a so-called "coverage gap." They have incomes above Medicaid eligibility limits, but they are below the lower limit for the marketplace premium tax credits, in which they could receive some kind of subsidy. In 2019, Garfield et al. noted that more than two million poor uninsured adults fall into that coverage gap. Furthermore, 76 percent in that coverage gap are adults without dependent children. The South was found to have higher numbers of poor, uninsured adults than in other regions, along with higher uninsured rates and more limited Medicaid eligibility than other regions, accounting for nine out of the fourteen states that opted not to expand Medicaid. "As a result, more than nine in 10 people in the coverage gap reside in the South," Garfield et al. said.

One of the factors that is often ignored in rhetoric about health care reforms is the amount of money that could be saved simply by ensuring that pregnant mothers have adequate prenatal care, preventative services are used with regularity, and health care screening becomes a part of affordable care. States that have implemented health care programs that provide for individual coverage have demonstrated clear gains from improving access to these types of services.

◆ Health Care and the Elderly

The American population is growing older every day, and this graying of the US population will have an impact on how health care resources are allocated, how health professionals address both short and long-term care scenarios, and how the workforce in the health care sector will meet the needs of a growing geriatric population. In the United States, the number of Americans over the age of sixty-five is anticipated to double from the current figure of approximately fifty million to nearly a hundred million by 2060 (Haseltine 2018). The United States is currently ranked among the top countries in the world for the elderly; there are, however, variations among this population when it comes to health care and quality of life (Haseltine 2018).

Narrowing this down further, the year 2035 is considered a major demographic turning point in the issue of aging in the United States (Meinert 2018). According to the US Census Bureau, by 2035, there will be 78 million people age sixty-five and older, versus 76.4 million under the age of eighteen. In other words, this means that the elderly population will outnumber children for the first time in US history, and this will lead to what Meinert dubbed "a unique set of public health challenges." Adding to the scenario is that not all seniors age the same. There is a longer life expectancy among foreign-born minorities, which has also contributed to the growth of the overall older adult population. Interestingly enough, foreign-born minorities tend to live longer than their US-born counterparts, meaning they spend more time in the category of "non-working, older adult."

Accommodating the needs of a diverse population, including different ethnicities, languages, and cultures, creates its own challenges for both health care and social work. The first thought that might come to mind, when mentioning "health care" and "elderly" in the same breath, is Medicare. After all, isn't Medicare considered the bellwether on which the entire US health care system should be based? Insurance coverage for all?

◆ Better Control of Costs?

Yes and no. In its more than fifty years of existence, Medicare has helped drive America's health care modernization, while providing a cushion between retired senior citizens and the increasing health care costs (Newkirk 2016). This has been helpful for women, especially older women who haven't received the same employment benefits as men. "As women have also always been much poorer than men, the poverty-lifting effects of Medicare were felt most along gender lines," Newkirk writes.

Then, there is the not-so-good news, according to the Commonwealth Fund's 20th International Health Policy survey, which indicated that Medicare beneficiaries tend to be sicker and to forgo medical care more often, due to costs, than their counterparts in Europe or Canada (Seegert 2017). In this survey, the United

States ranked at or near the bottom of many categories, including access, affordability, care timeliness, and care coordination. The study compared the US population of people sixty-five and older with their counterparts in Australia, Canada, France, Germany, the Netherlands, New Zealand, Norway, Sweden, Switzerland, and the United Kingdom. It was found that more than one in three (36 percent) Americans surveyed had multiple, chronic conditions. However, 23 percent of US seniors surveyed said they didn't go to a doctor when they were sick, get the recommended medical tests or procedures, or fill a needed prescription. The reasons? High costs. Yet in the UK, France, Norway, and Sweden, 5 percent or fewer seniors reported skipping needed care, due to costs.

Robin Osborn, vice president of the Commonwealth Fund's International Program in Health Policy and Practice Innovations, and lead author on the study, indicated that despite having Medicare (a version of universal coverage), older US adults are sicker and more economically vulnerable. "U.S. seniors struggle to afford care, and face more financial barriers to care than in the 10 other countries," Osborn said in a press conference.

This is because, similar to other insurance plans in the United States, Medicare's structure requires more out-of-pocket expenditures than health insurance in the other nations in the Commonwealth study. Twenty-two percent of US seniors spent $2,000 in out-of-pocket costs, such as co-pays, coinsurance, or prescription drugs. In the other countries (with the exception of Switzerland), fewer than 10 percent of seniors spent this much. Adding to the issue was that 25 percent of older US adults expressed concerns about having enough money to buy food and pay rent and utility bills, or had serious problems paying medical bills. In France, the UK, Norway, and Sweden, fewer than 5 percent of seniors indicated they struggled due to health care costs.

One issue, much as it is with poverty-level citizens, is economic vulnerability among seniors. Poverty, combined with unstable housing, social isolation, and mental health issues, are contributing to higher rates of chronic illness, poor health, and higher use of the health care system. Finally, the survey pointed out that "Medicare is not as generous as comparable insurance in other countries"; in addition, social and economic disparities are more prevalent in the United States than in the other nations surveyed.

One problem faced by Medicare in its current form is that it "doesn't seem to have the horsepower to accommodate the longer life spans and higher rates of poverty to anywhere near the point of gender equality" (Newkirk 2016). Basic Medicare doesn't provide dental care, hearing aids, nonmedically necessary foot care, long-term supports, or nursing homes, all of which can be problematic for older populations suffering from disabilities, chronic diseases, and dementia. Basic Medicare pays half of medical costs, though recipients can turn to Medicare Advantage plans and other private insurance providers for necessary services and to close the gap of out-of-pocket costs.

Still, the added costs above, plus co-payments/co-insurance, high drug prices, and other out-of-pocket costs can impact seniors and their ability to afford health care. It especially impacts older women, who are finding that Medicare isn't necessarily the silver bullet it was cut out to be. As such, care needs to be taken when discussing the benefits of Medicare for All, especially as Medicare, in its current form, isn't necessarily helping the senior population 100 percent.

◆ Shifting Costs to Consumers

For decades, many employers have used managed care plans, HMOs, PPOs, and other plans that integrated restrictions on the services that an individual could select, including the providers who could be used, as a basis for creating care while also maintaining cost-effectiveness. In recent years, the rising cost of health care has led employers to pass on the costs of health care to their employees (Reed et al. 2009). The increasing use of health savings accounts (HSAs) in conjunction with high-deductible health insurance plans has been viewed as one means of creating more effective responses to health insurance needs while also lowering overall costs.

Lee and Zapert (2005) assessed the impacts of the use of high-deductible health insurance plans in conjunction with, as well as separate from, the use of health savings accounts. One of the key aspects about this research was the attempt to determine whether individuals with high-deductible health insurance plans actually sought health care when needed, or if the presence of high deductibles was cost-prohibitive to ensuring access to health care. Approximately one-fourth of all insured individuals in the United States are insured using high-deductible health insurance plans. This places the responsibility of paying for a minimum of the first thousand dollars of care in the hands of the individuals who are insured, requiring considerable out-of-pocket expenses before any real benefits can be produced from the presence of health insurance.

While this may not have a major impact on individuals who have health issues, those who require the immediate payment of the thousand dollars and subsequent use of hundreds of thousands of dollars of insured services, the average family seeking to maintain cost savings in the presence of these plans could avoid basic services, from immunizations to pap smears and yearly physicals, as a result of the costs. I started out with the story of the Recchi family, which had to pay out thousands before a treatment plan could even be developed. While that scenario is an extreme case of out-of-pocket costs, a thousand dollars out of pocket can have huge consequences for a family that might assume its health insurance will cover costs.

Zapert's studies focused on early 2000s numbers. Fast-forward to the present, and we see that things haven't changed all that much. In fact, according to a study issued by the University of Southern California (USC), high-deductible health plans, touted for their money-saving potential, can greatly increase risk of high, out-of-pocket health care costs, especially among low-income Americans or those who are chronically ill (Gersema 2018). With earlier research defining excessive financial burden for consumers as spending more than 3 percent of their income on health issues, USC researchers found that the likelihood of financial trouble was higher for all enrollees on high-deductible plans, with more than one-half of low-income enrollees and more than one-third of those with chronic conditions facing excessive financial burden, after enrolling in a consumer-directed health plan. This was because enrollment in such a plan also increased the probability of high out-of-pocket spending on health care.

The results led the researchers to point out that low-income individuals, especially those with a chronic condition, who are employed with a company that switches to high-deductible insurance significantly increases the chances of facing a financial burden or a financial disaster. Why, then, are consumers selecting these higher-deductible plans? When the ACA required that everyone have health insurance, such plans at least came with low premiums. The same reason holds true, even with no mandate: higher-deductible plans carry lower premiums than those offered through traditional plans. While such plans do save money in the short term, it also shows that consumers on those plans don't increase their use of preventative care; this would, in turn, reduce overall costs.

It makes sense, as a higher deductible means there is less of a likelihood for individuals to seek medical services they might have to pay for on an already limited budget. Furthermore, researchers from the USC study noted that there isn't a reduction in use of unnecessary services under such plans. What ends up happening is that rather than seeking out preventative care early on, or obtaining treatment for an illness early on, those with high-deductible insurance plans wait until they are too sick to function.

Under such circumstances, by the time these patients do visit a health care provider, it will cost more to treat an illness, and that illness will likely require longer to cure. For example, a mammogram can aid in early breast cancer detection. However, if a woman's high-deductible insurance plan doesn't cover such a test, she might not be diagnosed until she ends up with Stage IV cancer, requiring a double mastectomy, weeks off from work, physical therapy, and prosthetics. This ends up as a large health care cost, which could have been avoided with a lower-deductible plan (or, rather, a better-thought-out health care system).

CHAPTER SIX: CAN HEALTH CARE REFORM WORK IN THE UNITED STATES?

"THE HISTORY OF AMERICAN HEALTH CARE REFORM HAS been filled with surprises," Dorn noted (2017). But Dorn and others point out, quite rightly, that health insurance is expensive because health care itself is expensive. Therefore, there is more to fixing the health care system than simply ensuring that every man, woman, and child in America has access to insurance. What is needed is help in reducing health care costs. The ACA was supposed to help with this; however, due to its patchwork nature, the legislation has actually meant some costs have spiraled out of control. The goal, instead, should be directed toward creating better health care consumers rather than pointing everyone toward high-value care, value-based insurance designs, and higher deductibles (Dorn 2017).

So is universal coverage or single-payer the answer? In truth, some version of both of these systems exists in the United States, and we'll take a look at how they operate. But first, we need to understand the difference between what is known as universal coverage and single-payer coverage.

◆ Clarifying Universal Coverage versus Single-Payer

"Universal coverage" and "single-payer" have been mentioned a great deal when it comes to reform of the US health care system. These terms tend to be used interchangeably, though both are very different, and they provide different options for different outcomes. Universal coverage refers to a health care system in which every individual has some kind of health insurance coverage (Montgomery 2019). There are currently approximately thirty-two countries with some form of universal health coverage. The United States, of course, does not have universal health coverage, as approximately 28.1 million Americans were without health insurance as of 2016. Canada, on the other hand, does have universal health coverage, through the government-run health care system. Incidentally, Canada's system does not provide coverage to undocumented immigrants. The ACA does not provide coverage to undocumented immigrants, either, despite what opponents of the act might suggest.

Meanwhile, a single-payer system is one in which a single entity——typically, the government—is 100 percent responsible for paying health care claims (Montgomery 2019). In the United States, the Veterans Health Administration provides an excellent example of a single-payer system; we'll examine the VHA in greater detail. Worldwide, seventeen countries offer a single-payer system, including Japan, the United Kingdom, and Spain. Medicaid, which is jointly funded by the federal government and state governments, is not single-payer, as the funding comes from two sources, rather than one.

The confusion between universal coverage and a single-payer

system is because these two can go often hand in hand. The reason is because a country's federal government is the most likely to administer and pay for a health care system that covers millions of people. Some countries, such as Denmark, France, and Australia, do operate a two-tier system, in which the government provides basic health care, while private insurance offers secondary coverage for those who can afford, and might want, a higher standard of care.

Then how does socialized medicine fit into the scenario? Unfortunately, opponents of health care reform in the United States might sling the "socialized" term around to strike fear into the hearts of others. Sen. Bernie Sanders (I-Vermont), the first to introduce the idea of Medicare for all, has been accused of promoting socialized medicine, but this isn't really true. In a socialized medical system, the government pays for health care and also oversees operations of hospitals and employs medical staff. Once again, the VHA is a good example of socialized medicine. Opponents of Medicare for All and similar programs like to point out what a mess the VHA is, but in actuality, it does the job, and does it well.

The UK's National Health Service is an example of a system in which the government pays for services, owns the hospitals, and employs the doctors and other health care providers. Meanwhile, Canada (which, once again, the more conservative dubs "socialized medicine") has a single-payer system with universal coverage, the hospitals are privately operated, and doctors aren't employed by the government (Montgomery 2019). In this situation, health care providers bill the government for services provided.

To summarize: Universal coverage ensures that everyone is covered by insurance. A single-payer system is when one entity (typically, a government) handles all health care; this is considered socialized medicine.

◆ Government-Funded Universal Coverage: Medicare

Medicare is a federal government program that provides health insurance to US residents who are sixty-five years and older (Introduction to Medicare 2019). Medicare is also open to US citizens who are under the age of sixty-five and receive Social Security Disability Insurance (or who are under sixty-five with end-stage renal disease). The program is run by the Centers for Medicare & Medicaid Services, a federal agency, and is paid for by Social Security and Medicare taxes paid on income. Also contributing to the funding are premiums paid on additional Medicare insurance and, in part, by the federal budget. Incidentally, Medicare coverage is only open to US citizens and permanent residents, and only if they have worked in the United States for forty quarters (which translates to ten years). Furthermore, only those who apply for Social Security benefits are eligible for Medicare.

Those who are Medicare-eligible can chose to receive their benefits from Original Medicare, a traditional fee-for-service program offered through the federal government, or Medicare Advantage, which is private insurance offered by companies that contract with the federal government (Introduction to Medicare 2019). Medicare Part D is a prescription and private drug plan.

Original Medicare covers subscribers for nearly all doctors and hospitals in the country, while Medicare Advantage Plans have network restrictions, based on the private insurance company that is being contracted with. However, Medicare Advantage can also provide additional benefits that Original Medicare doesn't cover, including routine vision or dental care (Introduction to Medicare 2019). Finally, there are Medicare Supplement plans (known as Medigap), which work alongside Original Medicare coverage to help with coverage gaps, such as out-of-pocket expenses. Medicare Part D and Medigap require additional payment from the subscriber.

The question revolves around the effectiveness of Medicare, which depends on who you talk to. Above, we mentioned that the poverty-stricken elderly might not do so well with Original Medicare, which might be all that this individual could afford. However, one study examined how health care spending, utilization, and price differ for adults with private insurance before and after they gain Medicare coverage at age sixty-five. The result was that "unadjusted spending per quarter for the services we analyzed fell sharply after entry into Medicare" versus costs for private insurance (Wallace and Song 2016, p. 867). In other words, compared to private insurance, costs were actually lower once an individual became a Medicare subscriber. The study was done in response to a belief that raising the age of entry into Medicare to sixty-seven years of age would reduce spending; this study demonstrated that the opposite is true. Costs would actually be higher if people delayed entry into Medicare.

However, when comparing administrative costs for private in-surance versus Medicare, there are some facts to consider. Let's get back to Bernie Sanders, who is basing his run for the 2020 presidency on a Medicare for All platform. He points out that private insurance companies in America spend between 12 and 18 percent, just on administrative costs (Tobias 2017). Meanwhile, Medicare spends just 2 percent on those same administrative costs. Technically, these numbers aren't wrong, but comparing Medicare to private insurance is a strictly apples-to-oranges exercise. This is because Medicare piggybacks off Social Security, meaning administrative costs, such as enrollment, payment, and keeping track of patients, are under the purview of Social Security, not the Centers for Medicare and Medicaid. "That's one of multiple reasons using the current administrative costs for Medicare wouldn't translate as cleanly if the entire population were to be covered," Politifact's Manuela Tobias wrote.

Then there is the fact that the average private insurer's overhead costs can run from 12.4 to 17.8 percent. However, the focus here is on averages (Tobias 2017). Administrative costs in the nongroup market are 20 percent, small-group market at 16 percent, and large-group market at 11 percent. Certainly, most of these costs are substantially higher than the Medicare administrative costs. However, private insurers do take responsibilities other than paying claims. For example, a private insurance company will determine if a particular medical procedure is necessary or whether that procedure can be done at a lesser cost, which is something that Medicare doesn't necessarily handle. In addition, administrative costs also go to marketing. Regardless of how someone feels about private insurance companies, they do need to compete for clients, which is something Medicare doesn't have to deal with.

When it comes to satisfaction with the system, the majority of older adults surveyed had positive opinions, and those younger than age sixty-five placed a great deal of value on the program (Brodie, Hamel, and Norton 2015). Furthermore, the majority of Americans surveyed think it works well; older adults enrolled in Medicare are more likely to rate their health insurance as "excellent" and more likely to indicate they are very satisfied with deductibles, co-pays, and choice of providers. Older adults with Medicare are also less likely to report problems paying medical bills in the past year, compared to younger adults with private insurance. However, a 2008 survey found that among people on Medicare, beneficiaries younger than age sixty-five (who are on Medicare because they have disabilities) were more likely than older adults to report problems with access and coverage.

Other surveys demonstrated a concern among the public about Medicare's financial future, due to the overall increase in US health care costs, an aging population, and declining worker-to-beneficiary ratio. Furthermore, many Americans worry that the program won't be there for them when they retire.

To summarize: It seems as though Medicare beneficiaries, at least the older ones, are happy with the program and indicate they receive adequate care without having to overpay. Furthermore, administrative costs do appear to be lower than that of private insurance; however, costs are measured differently. Finally, while administrative and health care costs are likely to be lower in a Medicare for All scenario, they aren't as low as Sanders and some of his proponents might assume they are.

The issue with Medicare, however, continues to be the out-of-pocket costs. While the program does cover certain health care expenses, there are others, such as prescriptions and dental care, that require supplemental Medicare or private insurance plans. Furthermore, as mentioned above, co-pays and deductibles still need to be paid on certain Medicare plans, which represents a hardship when it comes to lower-income seniors. So while Medicare seems to work for seniors, a proportion of that population is falling through the cracks; these are people who might not be able to afford the out-of-pocket costs.

◆ Socialized Medicine/Single-Payer System: The Veterans Administration

The Veterans Health Administration is a perfect example of socialized medicine; the US government runs the system's hospitals and clinics, and employs the health care providers working within it. Now, whether the VHA is effectively helping those who serve depends on who you talk to. Created from a law signed by Abraham Lincoln to establish a national soldiers and sailors asylum, the VHA has become the nation's "largest integrated health system ... [a] single-payer health system, owned, run and financed by the federal government" (O'Shea 2016). These days, the VHA provides everything to current and retired veterans and their families, including comprehensive inpatient and outpatient services in more than fourteen hundred facilities nationwide.

Since 2014 (and even beforehand), the VHA has been subject of intense scrutiny. In one report, it was estimated that as many as two hundred thirty-eight thousand veterans might have passed away before receiving any kind of care. Furthermore, go onto any social media website, and you'll find some kind of horror story taking place at some VHA clinic in some part of the country. The Heritage Foundation's John O'Shea, for one, points to the VHA and its parent, the Veterans Administration, as an organization with "a pattern of choosing reaction over reform." He explained that the rapid expansion of facilities to relieve overcrowding that took place during and after World War II led to overcapacity. Additionally, Congress expanded VA health benefits, first to veterans who didn't have service-connected injuries and eventually to spouses and children of disabled or deceased veterans.

O'Shea focused on the idea that while extending benefits, in and of itself, isn't bad, the current system hasn't been able to handle the increase in patient load. As such, his suggestions included enacting fiscally responsible reforms, providing appropriate services and out-sourcing, as necessary, and refocusing efforts on service-connected health care needs; in other words, "provide the best possible care to veterans dealing with injuries or illness received in the line of duty." In other words, in reading all of the negative press and focus on the VHA, one might come away with a sense that if the United States were to focus on a single-payer system, it would be a shambles. After all, if the federal government can't even care for its veterans properly, how can it be expected to handle the illnesses of the entire US population?

The answer is, it probably can't handle health care for the entire population, not as it is currently set up. And furthermore, for all of its problems and negative press, the VHA has its ardent supporters. One such supporter, US Army Air Defense Artillery Officer (Ret.) Dominick Tao, has sung the praises of the VHA, sharing with readers his story about a broken leg and his fear about how much repairs would cost. Researching emergency room and surgery costs on the internet told him that he could expect to be charged upwards of seventeen thousand dollars to get his leg fixed. Yet when all was said and done, as an honorably discharged veteran, Tao's cost for every-thing—X-rays, orthopedic specialist visits, medications, and even a knee scooter—was a grand total of eight dollars, through the VHA (Tao 2017). Tao noted that the rationale behind such discounted health care to its audience, service members, is clear: The Army knows that healthy soldiers are more effective soldiers (Tao 2017). "A national health-care system that treats all citizens this way may offer similar benefits," Tao noted.

What about the criticism of the VHA services that focuses on inefficiencies and long wait times? Tao indicated that the waits might actually not be all that bad. Furthermore, "if Anthem, Cigna or an-other large U.S. health-insurance company were subject to the same level of congressional scrutiny ... I'm not sure they'd fare much better" (Tao 2017). However, Anthem, Cigna, United Healthcare, and others aren't subject to that same level of congressional scrutiny. They are private insurance companies and, as such, don't necessarily have to list any kind of quality-oriented metrics.

Rosenberg (2016) agreed with Tao's assessment, pointing out that one reason why the long wait times have come under fire is because the VHA is a single system, which has standards and, yes, transparency. Transparency means that the VHA publishes prices for drugs, while using its buying power to negotiate good discounts on behalf of patients. This is something that private insurance com-panies, or even hospitals, don't do. The VHA also has clear standards regarding how often patients should get a specific test, such as a colo-noscopy, and follows those standards. Finally, the VHA has stated maximum wait times for different types of appointments; thirty days is the maximum for nonemergency care. If those wait times are longer, the VHA tracks those times and tries to find out why they are so long. Patients with private insurance might also have specialist wait times of thirty days or longer, but there is no safety net that tracks the reason for such wait times.

Delving into this topic further, a study conducted by the RAND Corp. noted that wait times at the VHA for new patient primary and specialty care tend to be shorter than wait times reported in "focused studies" of the private sector (Longman 2018). And in another study provided by the Commonwealth Fund, one in four Americans reported they had to wait six or more days for an appointment with their primary care physicians, even when they were sick or needed care (Longman 2018). In comparison, most VHA medical centers "now offer same-day urgent primary-care and mental-health-care appointments," *Newsday's* Longman said.

In addition, the VHA's centralized record keeping means that doctors know what other providers have done with their patient. The treatment comes from a single, fixed budget with no payment per procedure. Because of this, there's no incentive to order unnecessary, expensive tests on people who don't need them. In addition, there are no facilities fees, which can also cut back on extra bills and extraneous charges.

What about charges of slow claims processing? While the VHA is working hard to streamline its claims processing, "it is ultimately Congress that makes it so difficult for many veterans to get VA care," Longman commented. Due to laws that limit eligibility, veterans are required to show that they are either poor or suffer from a disability related to military service to qualify for both health care services and pension benefits (Longman 2018). Furthermore, a continued lack of funding to implement upgraded equipment continues to hamper this organization. Until this legislation is addressed by US lawmakers, claims will continue to clog up the VHA system.

Longman also busted the VHA subpar care myth. "Compared with the rest of the U.S. health-care system, V.A.'s performance is pretty impressive," he observed. However, opponents of the VHA and single-payer care scoff at this idea, claiming that the organization doesn't offer much in the way of choice when it comes to doctors or facilities. Longman doesn't disagree with this assessment. While practitioner choice is important so is "providing co-ordinated, high-quality, cost-effective care," which is what the VA does (Longman 2018).

The VHA is not a panacea when it comes to veterans' health care. The organization has its issues. However, part of the problem rests with Congress itself, both in funding and in legislation. Without upgraded technology, the VHA is floundering. So in a sense, it's a self-fulfilling prophecy. The VHA isn't doing as well as it could be because it doesn't have enough of the right resources. As such, this is a strike against universal coverage. Not the concept, but the fact that the federal government, as it currently stands, can't be counted on to deliver it.

◆ Health Care Reform by the States

With the federal government and Congress gridlocked over the ability to support, pass, and put into action meaningful health care reform, many states and municipalities have tried their own methods of universal and even single-payer systems. In many cases, these state and regional efforts are being studied to see how they might translate nationally. However, as of now, these efforts haven't led to a huge, resounding success. Below are some examples of these efforts:

◆ Massachusetts and Romneycare

Often called the prototype for the Affordable Care Act, Massachusetts' health care legislation, passed under the direction of Republican Governor Mitt Romney in 2006, was an attempt to move the state to universal health insurance coverage, with the goal of improving citizens' access to affordable, high-quality health care (Long, Skopec, Shelto, Nordahl, and Walsh 2016). After passage of the legislation, An Act Providing Access to Affordable, Quality, Accountable Health Care, statewide uninsurance rates dropped from 7.7 percent in 2006 to 3 percent in 2008; during the same period, the national uninsurance rates remained largely unchanged (Long et al. 2016). Though uninsurance rates did increase slightly during 2009–2013—likely due to the impacts of the Great Recession and continued increase in health insurance costs—uninsurance has remained at or below 50 percent.

While decreasing the number of uninsured is good news, as Long et al. (2016) point out, "coverage does not guarantee access to health care or access to affordable health care" (p. 1,633). Adults in Massachusetts continue to have difficulty finding health care providers and still have problems paying medical bills. Here are other factors from the Long et al. study: Gaps in coverage persist, especially among nonelderly adults. Uninsurance was particularly high for immigrants, minorities, those with less than a high school education, and those with family incomes at or below 138 percent of the poverty level.

Gaps in access and affordability persist. Though expansion of coverage led to improved access and greater affordability early on, those gains decreased, over time. In 2015, more than one-third of full-year insured adults reported going without some type of needed care, partly due to difficulty in finding providers who would see them or difficulty in getting timely appointments. Problems with access to care and affordability of care were most common for insured adults in fair or poor health and for those having lower family incomes. Long et al. concluded that while expanded coverage is a start, such coverage needs to reach eligible populations; furthermore, the coverage should also factor in access to affordable care.

A later study, conducted for 2018, found that while the state has been highly successful in maintaining near-universal health insurance coverage, "the high levels of health insurance coverage did not guarantee access to health care or the affordability of care" (Long and Aaron 2018). Close to half the adults surveyed reported difficulty in obtaining health care over the past year, with close to 40 percent going without needed health care. Low- to moderate-income adults were more likely than low-income or higher-income adults to have problems paying medical bills. "As was true of earlier rounds of the MHRS [Massachusetts Health Reform Survey], the 2018 MHRS is a reminder that the goals of health care reform are not achieved by simply reducing the number of people in Massachusetts who are uninsured," the researchers concluded. They added that strategies are needed to improve access to care, while reducing the burden of health care costs.

Added to this, the individual marketplaces haven't lived up to expectations (Hacker 2018). The enrollment of twelve million people is approximately half of what the nonpartisan Congressional Budget Office projected when the law passed back in 2006. And, as mentioned above, those who have enrolled have been less healthy than expected, which has, in turn, driven up premiums. It's easy to extrapolate Romneycare to Obamacare, as the results, in many cases, seem to be the same. Insurance coverage isn't the same as access to quality health care. If a system is overwhelmed by less healthy people, premiums increase, something that is happening with the Affordable Care Act.

◆ Vermont and the Single-Payer, Universal Health Care System

Sen. Bernie Sanders's home state is Vermont. And some years ago, Vermont became ground zero for universal coverage, with a single-payer health care focus. On May 26, 2011, Act 48 passed in Vermont, spearheaded by then-Vermont Governor Peter Shulmin. The plan called for a government-financed system, called Green Mountain Care, to provide universal coverage. Green Mountain Care, itself, was an answer to disappointment concerning the ACA's compromises with the private insurance industry.

A study for the state, conducted by Harvard health economist William Hsaio, focused on incrementally moving the state toward a public-private system, financed through a 14.2 percent payroll tax: employers would pay 10.6 percent, while employees would be responsible for the remaining 3.6 percent. The public-private partnership was developed, in part, to tamp down fears of a wholly government-run program. Furthermore, the plan would be implemented incrementally alongside the ACA rollout, to avoid legal battles with the government.

While this plan did include some of the features of reform recommendations from the Hsiao report, it ended up being vague on other specific details. One of those vague details was how the system would be financed. Shulman and his staff felt that including a specific financing plan in the initial bill would leave it open to attacks from opponents, possibly killing the bill. The bill, therefore, incorporated delayed implementation, with those supporting the bill reasoning that financing decisions could be postponed until after the bill was passed. It was this procrastination that, in part, ended up dooming the legislation.

Another problem with the bill had to do with Green Mountain Care itself, specifically, the five-person board appointed to oversee the design of the plan. The board was responsible for addressing major factors that included the cost of health care, benefits, coverage, and premiums. Furthermore, the board functioned as a regulatory public service entity, with a quasi-judicial policymaking role, versus the public-private partnership suggested in Hsiao's report. Board members ultimately made decisions concerning hospital budgets and insurance rates, adding a level of unnecessary bureaucracy.

Meanwhile, as Green Mountain Care's 2017 launch date drew near, other issues came up; there was still no specific focus on how the plan would be financed. Shulman's original thought had been to gradually increase Medicaid spending by 3 percent from 2012 to 2017 and use that money to set up the program's infrastructure. The state received $1.17 in matching funds from the federal government for every $1.00 it put into the program. However, the state economy wasn't growing as quickly as originally thought, and it was found that the state couldn't afford those 3 percent increases or match funds that would come alongside those increases.

Then there was Shulman himself, who couldn't keep his hands off the bill. In one case, the governor and state legislature responded to lobbying by business interests and adjusted the law to allow non-residents working within the state to join Green Mountain Care. This, of course, meant a higher number of people would need to be covered. Other changes raised the expected portion of medical costs covered by the plan, rather than through out-of-pocket spending, from 87 to 94 percent, while eliminating state taxes on health care providers. The end result was an increase in the program's costs and a decrease in the revenue necessary to pay for it.

Finally, while Shulman and his team worked hard on developing Green Mountain Care's policy between 2011 and 2014, they forgot to educate the public about what, exactly, the bill would mean to those covered and how it would impact people's lives. This, in turn, led to confusion about the plan, especially when Vermont Health Connect, the state's ACA health insurance website, went live in October 2013. Much like what happened with the ACA website rollout, Healthcare.gov, Vermont Health Connect was plagued by issues. It took Shulman a year to fix the issues (before shutting the site down for repairs in September 2014), which eroded the public's trust in the government's ability to handle health care.

By the end of 2014, Shulman no longer had confidence in the reform effort. After barely squeaking through to win the governorship against a candidate who actively campaigned against a single-payer system, Shulman officially and publicly withdrew the plan in December 2014. While three studies focused on Green Mountain Care's viability indicated the state would save money by implementing the program, the size of the taxes needed to support the program would have been "a political nonstarter without a sustained effort to educate the public." In addition, by putting off how the program would be financed until well after the bill had passed, the government missed a chance to build a constituency that would support the idea that Green Mountain Care's benefits would outweigh the costs.

The Vermont government didn't have answers for issues that included the higher-than-expected payroll tax or even issues dealing with Vermont Health Connect. This scenario gave the impression that the government was floundering when it came to health care issues. In addition, the plan was unpopular with hospitals and insurance companies; it forced hospitals to receive Medicare-like payments and undergo pay cuts, while pretty much abolishing private insurance plans. Once again, it wasn't the single-payer concept or the idea of universal coverage that doomed the plan. Rather, it was the ham-fisted way in which everything was rolled out.

◆ California's (Attempted) Move to a Universal System

Gavin Newsom was elected governor of the state of California, partly because of his promise to bring universal health care to its residents (Thompson 2018). And Senate Bill 562 was introduced in an attempt to replace California's patchwork insurance system with a single-payer model, in which the state would finance health care for all residents. That bill stalled in the senate and eventually died.

However, even with Newsom's promises to support single-payer coverage, experts point out that there are several issues to resolve; one of those issues involves collaboration with the federal government. This would require changes in US law, as well as federal government waivers that would allow the state to redirect federal health care funds, and given that the Trump administration isn't a fan of the Golden State at this time, this type of collaboration is very unlikely. Furthermore, while a universal system eliminating premiums would eventually provide savings to taxpayers, two studies conducted in 2017 noted that implementation of such a system would require new taxes ranging from $100 billion to $200 billion.

If that weren't bad enough, the additional complication is Proposition 98, which was passed in 1988. The proposition requires that 40 percent of the state's general revenue go toward K–12 school funding. This could be a problem if the state raises taxes for a single-payer system, as a good chunk of that funding would go toward education. Fixing the conflict would require a statewide ballot protecting health care taxes from the requirements of Proposition 98.

Finally, affordability issues plague Covered California, the health care exchange that was created after the passage of the ACA. Laurel Lucia, director of the Health Care Program at the University of California-Berkeley's Labor Center, notes that plenty of people in the state don't have job-based coverage and are struggling to afford individual coverage. This is a particular problem in California, she added, as the ACA doesn't adjust subsidies based on cost of living. Still, the proposed expansion of Medi-Cal (California's Medicaid) to undocumented adults, combined with increased state subsidies, could help the state provide universal health care, at the very least.

So far, however, while a single-payer system or universal health care are supported by many, it doesn't seem to be budging much from the idea stage. There are many thoughts and cost estimates, as well as concerns. However, while Newsome did offer a sweeping health care reform policy on his first day in office as governor, right now, nothing much has changed. California is incrementally moving toward the idea of universal coverage, but it's too soon to determine if this will actually happen.

◆ New York City's Universal Health Insurance Program

In January 2019, New York City Mayor Michael de Blasio announced a $100 million health insurance program to cover six hundred thousand uninsured metro residents (Cherelus 2019). The plan focuses on those unable to afford coverage, as well as undocumented immigrants. Dubbed the NYC Care plan, de Blasio indicated it would be funded without tax increases as an expansion of the city's existing MetroPlus plan. That plan covers hospital bills for low-income residents. NYC Care provides insurance for doctors' visits outside of hospitals; health experts suggest that regular medical visits can cut down on costly hospital stays.

NYC Care will be officially launched in the Bronx in summer 2019 and will expand across the entire city by 2021. Mayor de Blasio indicated that all services would be affordable on a sliding scale for those who can pay a portion of the costs. Those unable to afford the cost will receive free health care. Again, it is too soon to see how, or if, NYC Care will work. And while there has been a push in the New York state legislature to adopt universal health care, Governor Andrew Cuomo and some Democrats in Albany suggest the costs of such a plan could double the state's $170 billion budget and require new taxes (Spector 2019).

◆ Discussion

The above focused on working systems of universal coverage and single-payer systems currently in operation in the United States. Sadly, the two attempts at health care reform that actually made it through legislation haven't been too positive in terms of effectiveness. Vermont's plan fell short, primarily because it was vague and opaque. And while most of the Massachusetts population is insured, access to health care is the main problem there.

On a national level, Medicare and the VHA seem to be effective in terms of delivery of care and cost controls, even though these two systems have their problems, and they haven't been effective for everyone. But these systems cover only a part of the population, and questions remain as to whether extrapolating either or both (assuming legislation could even get through Congress) is possible.

CHAPTER SEVEN: COUNTRY-TO-COUNTRY HEALTH CARE COMPARISONS

WHEN DISCUSSING HEALTH CARE REFORM, THE DISCUS-
sion inevitably turns to how US health care coverage compares to
that of other countries. This chapter will delve into detail on these
comparisons, but first, an overview.

One study, conducted by Selberg et al. (2018), measured whether
health care value has increased in the United States over the past
quarter-century. The results were a mixed bag; between 1991 and
2016, life expectancy increased by 3.1 years to 78.6 years, which
was a 4 percent improvement. At the same time, disease burden
improved by 12 percent, meaning fewer years living with disabilities
and fewer years of life lost to premature death. The not-so-good news
was that the increased life expectancy and reduced disease burden
didn't keep pace with a 40 percent increase in GDP health care consumption (Selberg et al. 2018).

Basically, over the past twenty-five years, nations similar in size
and wealth to the United States generated an average life expectancy
improvement of 5.2 years, or a 7 percent increase, compared to a

4 percent improvement in America. Furthermore, disease burden in these countries improved by 22 percent, versus the 12 percent reported in the United States. On average, "comparable countries spend under two thirds [60 percent] of what the U.S. spends on healthcare, relative to GDP," Selberg et al. noted. The researchers concluded their study by pointing out that by comparing health care systems of other countries, the United States has plenty of room and opportunity to increase efficiencies and improve life expectancies, while reducing disease burden.

Furthermore, "the data appear to support the contention that U.S. healthcare does have a higher threshold to overcome with regard to socioeconomic factors and lower investment in social services," Selberg and his colleagues noted. This isn't exactly shocking; it's something we pointed out earlier.

The difficulty, however, in any kind of honest comparisons with health care systems from other countries is, rhetoric tends to bury the reality of the situation. For example, people aren't collapsing and dying in the United Kingdom because the wait time to see a doctor can be up to six months (which actually isn't true, but this is part of the rhetoric). However, long wait times can be the norm in the UK. Then again, long wait times are also part of the US health care system. To gain a better perspective on costs and outcomes, it is instructive to take a nonbiased look at how the US health care system compares to that of other industrialized nations. We will focus on health care in three countries: Canada, Germany, and the United Kingdom.

◆ Canada

Depending on who you talk to, the Canadian health care system is either the greatest in the world or the worst. Stories coming out of the country north of the border range from ill people walking into hospitals, being treated, and paying next to nothing, to patients having to wait for months to see a doctor for treatment.

As with most things, the reality is somewhere in between. Yes, basic care (i.e., care provided by physicians and hospitals) is free; no premiums, deductibles, or co-payments are required (O'Neill and O'Neill 2007). However, other services, such as dental, prescription drugs, and health care above the basic services, need to be paid either through private insurance or out of pocket. Canada's national health insurance (NHI) program is a government-run health insurance system that covers the entire population with a well-defined medical benefits package (Ridic, Gleason, and Ridic 2012). Health insurance coverage is universal, with general taxes financing NHI through a single-payer system.

Physician choice is unlimited, and there are no co-payments; physicians receive payments on a negotiated fee for service, while hospitals receive global budget payments. In other words, reimbursement takes place between the public insurer (the government) and the provider (Ridic, Gleason, and Ridic 2012). We will discuss global budgets later on; this is a method used by third-party payers to control costs by establishing total spending limits for services, over a specific period of time. These global budgets help with cost control.

Canada finances basic health care through six provincial payers (Holland 2017). While its Medicare system (not the same as the US

Medicare system) does provide good, basic coverage, approximately two in three Canadians must purchase supplemental insurance for prescription drugs, vision care, and dental health. Approximately 30 percent of all Canadian health care is financed through the private sector.

It's interesting that in the mid-twentieth century, the United States and Canada had similar health care systems, with both offering fee-for-service plans and insurance. In the 1940s, some Canadian provinces went one step further and introduced compulsory health insurance. Immediately following World War II, the province of Saskatchewan set up a hospitalization plan (Ridic, Gleason, and Ridic 2012). This plan created a regional system of hospitals: local hospitals for primary care, district hospitals for more complex, cases and base hospitals that handled more difficult cases. In 1956, Canada's federal parliament enacted the Hospital and Diagnostic Services Act, which provided a groundwork for a national system of hospital insurance. By 1971, Canada had a health insurance plan, which provided coverage for both hospitalization and physician services. In the 1970s, both the United States and Canada spent 7.5 percent of their GDP on health care. As has been pointed out already, the US GDP is well beyond that 7.5 percent. Meanwhile, overall health spending in Canada is at 11.3 percent.

While health care costs are less than those in the United States, the wait times for certain procedures are high. Nationwide (as of 2012), the average wait time for treatment is 13.3 weeks, and if care required diagnostic imaging, the waiting times are even longer. Some of the treatment delays are creating problems for certain segments of the population, particularly the elderly, who can't get reasonable access to care such as hip replacements, cardiovascular surgery, or cataract surgery.

Furthermore, some studies have found Canadian health care deficient in areas such as angioplasty, cardiac catheterization, and intensive care. In addition, Ridic et al. (2012) and O'Neill and O'Neill (2007) point out that whenever anything is provided for free (such as health care), both demand and spending increase. Resource allocations tend to become more inefficient over time, with the government forced to either increase revenue or drop services.

During the 1990s, when the federal government in Canada cut back block amounts given to the provinces, shortages in health care deliveries developed, and health care rationing became more widespread. During the 2000s, many of the provincial health plans dropped services from the list of approved, medically necessary treatments in order to reduce costs. The situation in Canada is that the so-called free health care does lead to longer wait times or unavailable services (and, in response, unmet needs). Meanwhile, in the United States, costs are more often linked to unmet needs.

Finally, as government regulators make resource allocation decisions when it comes to health care, this control extends to capital investment in hospitals, specialty mix of medical practitioners, and the location of medical graduates and high-tech equipment. In 1997, Canada had fifty-two MRIs, which is one for every 572,000 citizens; contrast this to the 2,046 MRIs in the United States (one for every 130,800 Americans). On the other side of the coin, the US health care system tends to be overly reliant on tests; perhaps all of those MRIs aren't really needed.

It's instructive to understand, however, that even with the wait time to see health care providers and the concept of rationing, most Canadians support their version of health care and actually like it. Basically, the medical care system, with all of its faults, provides its residents with access to necessary hospital and physician services, all at a fraction of the cost of the US system. In addition, the administrative aspect of the system is easier; rather than receiving multiple bills to treat a single illness, Canadians receive either no bill or a single bill for treatment. The administrative costs are far less.

◆ Germany

When discussions about health care come up in the United States, the two countries it is compared to are the United Kingdom and Canada. However, Germany offers an interesting look into the effectiveness of socialized medicine. Today's German health care system can be found from mutual aid societies formed in the early nineteenth century. When Otto von Bismarck became Germany's first chancellor in 1871, hundreds of sickness insurance funds were already in existence; Bismarck expanded those benefit societies to cover all workers in low-wage occupations. The Sickness Insurance Act was passed in the late nineteenth century.

For more than a century, virtually all of the German population have had access to health care, and all individuals are required, by law, to have access to health insurance. Those earning less than $35,000 (as of the mid-1990s) are required to join one of the sickness funds for their health care coverage. These sickness funds are private, nonprofit insurance companies that collect premiums from employees and employers to pay for the coverage. Individual health insurance premiums for workers are calculated on the basis of income, rather than age or number of dependents. The sickness funds pay providers directly for services provided to members, at rates that are negotiated with individual hospitals.

Furthermore, these funds, by law, are required to provide a comprehensive set of benefits. Germany's single-payer system has 125 nonprofit insurers that participate in one national exchange (Holland 2017). Approximately 10 percent of Germans—the wealthiest ones—actually opt out of the national system and purchase their health care from for-profit insurance companies. When it comes to government involvement, the central government passes legislation on policy and jurisdiction, whereas state governments take on responsibility for managing state hospitals and supervising the sickness funds and physician associations. The local governments oversee local hospitals and public health programs; it's a highly decentralized system.

On the positive side, Germany has succeeded in controlling health care costs because of the framework of its health care system. By linking medical expenditures to sickness fund members' income, however, the success depends on the continued growth in wages and salaries, as well as negotiations between sickness funds and medical practitioners. On the other side of the coin, the cost-containment measures have taken a bite out of physicians' incomes. While they aren't hurting, they aren't as highly paid as elsewhere (such as the United States).

Additionally, the German system, as it currently stands, could be considered unsustainable. Much like Canada, German patients have little to no incentive to limit their demand for, and consumption of, health care services. Nor do health care providers have any incentive to limit supply, and the ability of the system to control costs depends on relative bargaining power between the sickness funds and medical providers.

Finally, the system doesn't use resources efficiently, as incentives promote the use of invasive acute care procedures, while discouraging the provision of personal services. Germans visit their doctors more often, the average hospital length of stay is longer, and doctors prescribe more prescription drugs. Furthermore, the system is likely to be more burdened by an aging population, which could put additional pressure on the supply and health care delivery.

However, similar to Canadian citizens and their health care system, German residents like their health care. Part of the reason is because wealthy Germans do have access to a private insurance safety valve, if needed. Furthermore, German culture is one of social solidarity, a belief that the government is responsible when it comes to providing a wide range of social benefits to all citizens, ranging from old-age pensions, to unemployment insurance, to health care. Still, in one survey, 48 percent of Germans surveyed indicated that their health care system either needed fundamental changes or should be rebuilt completely.

◆ The United Kingdom

The main issues to understand about health care in the United Kingdom is that it is free at the point of use, to anyone who needs it. No paperwork is required, no bills are received, and no one in the UK goes bankrupt through medical costs. The health care itself, however, is just okay.

The United Kingdom's health care system is overseen by the National Health Service (NHS), a government-funded system that provides free-of-charge care to UK residents (Thorlby and Arora 2017). Those eligible for NHS have access to care without discrimination and are guaranteed care within certain time limits (such as emergency and planned hospital care). The NHS provides or pays for preventative health care services, which include screening, immunizations, vaccination programs, inpatient/outpatient hospital care, physician services, prescriptions, clinically necessary dental care, mental health care, some eye care, palliative care, and some long-term care, which includes after-stroke care and home visits by community-based nurses.

While the Department of Health oversees the overall national health care system, the system's day-to-day operations rest within NHS England, which manages the health care budget, oversees 209 local clinical commissioning groups (CCGs), and makes sure that objectives listed in an annual mandate by the secretary of state for health are met. Local government authorities take charge of public health budgets; these authorities, in turn, are required to host "health and well-being boards" to improve coordination of local services, while reducing health disparities.

These local boards also determine the volume and scope of health care, but the NHS constitution indicates that patients have a right to drugs or treatment approved in technology appraisals, carried out by the National Institute of Health and Clinical Excellence (NICE), as long as this is recommended by a physician or clinician. For drugs or treatments NICE doesn't approve, the CCGs are responsible for making what is termed "rational, evidence-based decisions." The majority of funding for the NHS comes from taxation, with additional funds coming from a payroll tax. Income is also received from co-payments, people using NHS services as private patients, and other small sources.

Health care coverage in the UK is universal; residents in England are entitled to mostly free care at point of use; so are nonresidents who have a European Health Insurance card. Non-European visitors or undocumented immigrants can be treated for free in emergency departments. Still, an estimated 10.5 percent of the UK population has private, voluntary insurance; this offers faster and more convenient access to care, especially when it comes to elective hospital procedures. Furthermore, while care is generally free, limited cost-sharing arrangements are in place for publicly covered services.

Outpatient prescription drugs are subject to a co-payment, while drugs prescribed in NHS hospitals are free. Dentistry services are subject to co-payments, with charges set nationally by the Department of Health. Those exempt from prescription drug co-payments include children ages fifteen and under, and full-time students aged sixteen to nineteen. People age sixty and older, as well as those with low incomes, pregnant women, those who have given birth in the past twelve months, and people with cancer are also exempt from co-payment requirements. Those requiring large amounts of prescription drugs can acquire prepayment certificates costing $42 (USD) for three months and $150 (USD) for twelve months.

Primary care is delivered through general practitioners, who are also gatekeepers for secondary, or specialized, care. These general practices are normally the patients' first point of contact; patients are required to register with a local practice of their choice. This is where some cracks in the system start to emerge; GP choice is eliminated, as many practices are full and don't accept new patients. In some areas, however, walk-in centers do offer primary care services, for which registration isn't required.

Most general practices employ other health care workers, including nurses, and the practices themselves are moving from independent, solo entities to networked practices. These in turn, include multipractice organizations, consisting of specialists, pharmacists, and social workers. Approximately 56 percent of practices operate under national General Medical Services contracts, which are negotiated between the government and the British Medical Association. Payment is provided with a mix of capitation to cover essential services, optional fee-for-service payments for additional services, and an optimal performance-related scheme; capitation is based on local levels of morbidity and mortality, as well as age and gender, along with patient list turnover and market-forces factors for staff costs, compared with those of other practices. Performance bonuses are provided on evidence-based clinical intervention and chronic illness care coordination.

Along these lines, most of the practices are reimbursed monthly for services they deliver, based on data that is extracted from the electronic records of patients. Some of the practices are required to enter data manually for patients screened or treated for other services that qualify for additional payments; these, in turn, are collected and validated by NHS England. Publicly owned hospitals are organized as NHS trusts that are directly accountable to the Department of Health or as foundation trusts regulated by another organization, NHS Improvement. These hospitals contract with local CCGs to provide services and are reimbursed at nationally determined diagnosis-related group (DRG) rates, which include medical staff costs.

The United Kingdom also has more than five hundred private hospitals and between five and six hundred private clinics. These institutions offer treatments that either are not offered through the NHS or require longer wait times. However, these facilities typically don't have emergency, trauma, or intensive-care components. While private providers must be registered with the Care Quality Commission and NHS Improvement, their charges are not regulated, and there are no public subsidies involved.

NHS costs are contained through a global budget, rather than through direct constraints on supply or patient cost-sharing. The CCGs are allocated funds by NHS England and are expected to achieve a balanced budget each year. There has been, however, a mismatch between funding and demand and the cost of providing services, leading to a $5.3 billion (USD) deficit for 2015–2016 (the most recent metrics available). While some savings targets are being met, financial pressure on the NHS is leading to a deterioration in quality of care and increased waiting times. In recent years, NHS Improvement put a program into place to help hospital providers boost savings by improving staff efficiencies, as well as purchasing of drugs and medical equipment more cost-effectively and providing better facilities management.

Added to the problem is that since the financial crisis of 2008, the UK has been taking in less tax revenue and has had to cut spending (Frayer 2018). While the government's expenditure on the NHS continues growing, it has done so at a slower pace than in previous years. Prescriptions are being rationed, while thousands of elective surgeries have been postponed. Wait times at emergency rooms are also on the rise. As is what is happening in other countries, people are living longer and are having fewer children, and with older people requiring more expensive care, it is putting stress on the health care system. It will also be interesting to see what happens to the UK economy and, through it, the country's health care system, as the country continues to figure out ways in which it departs the European Union as a trading partner, due to Brexit.

However, a protest in early 2018 on Downing Street in London prompted President Donald Trump to say that British health care is "going broke and not working." This, of course, prompted those in the UK to reply that, for all of its troubles, the NHS is far better than the health care being offered in the United States. As such, while the NHS does have its problems, UK residents are very proud of it and are proud of the health care coverage they receive through it.

With the above descriptions of health care systems in the different countries in mind, what follows are health status dashboards comparing the four countries, based on data from Organization for Economic Co-operation and Development (OECD):

◆ Health Status

Life Expectancy (Male)
Life Expectancy (Female)
Ischemic Mortality
(Per 100,000)
Dementia
(Per 1,000)

◆ Canada

79.6

83.8

93

13

◆ Germany

78.3

83.1

106

20.2

◆ United Kingdom

79.2

82.8

98

17.1

◆ United States

76.3

81.2

113

11.6

While all of the above are within range of the OECD average (with the exception being dementia prevalence in Germany, which is worse than the OECD average), the United States has, on average, lower life expectancy among both males and females, and a higher rate of ischemic mortality, meaning more people in the United States are likely to die from the result of a stroke or heart attack.

◆ **Risk Factors for Health**

% of Population that Smokes Daily
Liters per Capita of Alcohol Consumed Annually
Obesity
% of Population with BMI > 30

◆ **Canada**

14.0
8.1
25.8

◆ **Germany**

20.9
11.0
23.6

◆ **United Kingdom**

16.1

9.5

26.9

◆ **United States**

11.4

8.8

38.2

The percentage of the US population that smokes and drinks is less than those of the three other countries. However, a greater percentage of the population—close to 40 percent—is considered obese. Those who are obese have a greater incidence of chronic diseases, which would include diabetes, heart disease, and stroke. And, as mentioned above, more people in the United States die from heart attacks and stroke than in the other three countries.

◆ **Access to Care**

% of Population Covered by Insurance

Share of Out-of-Pocket Costs (% of Household Consumption)

Consultations Skipped Due to Cost (per 100)

◆ **Canada**

100

2.2

6.6

◆ **Germany**

100

1.8

2.6

◆ **United Kingdom**

100

1.5

4.2

◆ **United States**

90.9

2.5

22.3

The above tells the story that could support a Medicare for All type of plan. Whereas citizens in the other three countries have 100 percent insurance coverage, the United States is well below the

OCED average at just under 91 percent. Furthermore, Americans pays a higher share of out-of-pocket costs (as a percentage of household consumption). Even worse is the number of patients, per 100, that skip consultations or appointments because they can't afford them. Close to one-quarter of the US population is not receiving the care it needs, simply because getting that care is too costly.

◆ Health Care Resources

Health Care Expenditure (Per Capita)
Doctors per Capita (1,000)
Nurses per Capita (1,000)
Beds per Capita (1,000)

◆ Canada

$4,753
2.7
9.9
2.6

◆ Germany

$5,551
4.1
13.3
8.1

◆ **United Kingdom**

$4,192

2.8

7.9

2.6

◆ **United States**

$9,892

2.6

11.3

2.8

In reference to the above, we've already pointed out several times that US health care is among the most expensive among industrialized societies. What is interesting with the above metrics, however, is that even countries practicing rationed health care seem to have similar numbers of resources. For example, Canada spends far less, per capita, on health care than does the United States yet has a similar number of doctors per capita as its neighbors to the south. The same is true when it comes to hospital beds. This is not to suggest that the rationed health care offered in Canada and the UK doesn't have its problems. What it does indicate, however, is that US expenditures are far higher than those from the other countries, with not a whole lot to really show for it. The available resources seem to be similar across the countries. What the above shows is that there is no such thing as a perfect health care system.

In addition, a study published in the *Journal of the American Medical Association* in March 2018 demonstrated that when it came to health care utilization, the United States didn't differ substantially from other high-income nations (Papanicolas, Woskie, and Jha 2018). In this study, researchers compared US health care structural capacity and utilization with ten other high-income countries (including Australia, Canada, France, Germany, and the United Kingdom). The researchers' goal wasn't so much to determine that Americans spend more, per capita, on health care than other nations; this is an already known fact. Rather, the researchers were more focused on explaining the differences in expenditures.

To come to their conclusion, the researchers analyzed comparative data on general health income spending, then focused on inputs (such as labor costs and structural capacity). They also analyzed outputs, or rather, access, utilization, patient experience, and quality of care, along with demographic differences, risk factors, and disease prevalence. Some of the results were interesting. While the United States ranked below the mean when it came to total social spending, it wasn't an outlier. Social spending focuses on spending on old age, incapacity, labor market, education, family, and housing. As we saw above, the United States had the highest percentage of overweight/obese adults but relatively low smoking rates, with the drinking age and unemployment rates both close to the mean values of the other ten countries.

Again, unsurprisingly, the United States consistently had the poorest population health outcomes and the lowest life expectancies, though there was a huge variability of life expectancies across the fifty states. The United States did have the highest infant, neonatal, and maternal mortality rates. However, when adjusting neonatal mortality to exclude deaths of infants born weighing less than 1,000 grams, America actually ranked fifth, relative to other countries, with 1.61 deaths per 1,000 live births. The mean was 1.70 deaths per live births for all eleven countries.

The US physician workforce was lower than the mean of a hundred countries (at 2.6 per 1,000 population, versus the 3.3 per 1,000 population mean); the proportion of physicians who were primary care doctors was the same as the mean of all eleven countries. The kicker here was that out of the countries surveyed, the United States had the highest level of administrative burden, which probably shouldn't be any surprise. Physicians in America reported having a higher level of administrative burden than the mean of the eleven countries, though the burden was high in all insurance-based systems.

Among the eleven countries, the United States also had the highest pharmaceutical spending per capita, at $1,443; this eclipsed Switzerland ($939) and the mean of $749 for all eleven countries. And finally, when examining health care access, America had the most inequitable access to physicians, when adjusted for need. In focusing on their conclusions, the researchers didn't blame under-investment in social programs, fee-for-service, defensive medicine, or overutilization for the higher cost of US health care. Rather, the researchers pointed to the prices themselves, specifically, hospital and physician prices, pharmaceuticals, and diagnostic tests, "which likely also affected access to care."

In other words, a focus on utilization alone won't reduce that spending gap between the United States and other high-wealth countries; the effort, instead, should focus on an effort to reduce prices and administrative costs. In other words, simply insuring everyone won't reduce costs as much as directly targeting the reasons for those continued costs might.

This chapter examined health care systems of other industrialized Western countries and showed that there is no such thing as a perfect system. Universal health care (as practiced by Canada and Germany) and a single-payer system (in the United Kingdom) have their flaws. But then again, so does the US health care system. There are wait times to see physicians in the United States. In addition, there are high costs, confusing out-of-pocket expenses, and huge administrative burdens. While Canada's, or the UK's solution might not be the answer in the United States, it is a good idea to take a careful, considerate look at these systems, rather than buying into the rhetoric.

CHAPTER EIGHT: THE POLITICS OF HEALTH CARE: DEMOCRATIC CANDIDATES

THE REPUBLICANS' FAILURE TO ERADICATE OBAMACARE isn't likely to be repeated by the Democrats, should they retake Congress and the presidency in 2020. This is because plans are already under way, and bills already introduced, to at least address the health care situation. The issue, as it continues to be, is how far such legislation will go through Congress before getting shot down.

In February 2019, Representative Pramila Jayapal (D-Washington) introduced a sweeping Medicare for All bill, that would create a single-payer, government-funded health care program within two years (Pramuk 2019). The plan would eliminate the sixty-five-year-old threshold for Medicare eligibility; wouldn't charge co-pays, premiums, or deductibles; and would cover prescription drugs, vision, dental, mental health, and maternal care, among other things. The plan, with its more than a hundred co-sponsors (all Democrats), was introduced during a time in which Republican efforts to repeal the Affordable Care Act have, for the most part, failed.

Needless to say, the bill has attracted backlash from Republicans, who consider it to be a "socialist idea." There are also Democrats who want to see health care reformed in more incremental steps, such as a Medicare or Medicaid buy-in. Regardless of where the bill goes, with the 2020 elections looming, health care is once again front and center. With more Democrats jumping into the race, what is also prevalent is their focus on reforming health care. We'll look at the plans of a few of the front-runners.

◆ Bernie Sanders: Medicare for All

Bernie Sanders, the independent senator from Vermont, has been making news, for years, with his idea of Medicare for All, in which all US residents are covered, with no co-pays or deductibles for medical services (Sanders 2018). This plan would be paid for by having employers pay a 7.5 percent income-based premium, increasing household taxes by 4 percent (income-based), and installing a more progressive personal income tax. Other ways to fund this system would include making the state tax more progressive, establishing a wealth tax on the top 0.1 percent, and imposing a fee on large financial institutions.

According to a George Mason University study, the Sanders plan would boost government health spending by $32.6 trillion over a ten-year period, which would also require "historic tax hikes" (Alonso-Zaldivar 2018). However, it has also been noted that US health care costs are trending at about the same level (Pauley and Field 2019). Additionally, the idea has support among the rank-and-file Democrats, with polls indicating that the plan appeals to many independent voters as well.

The study also found that the plan "would reap substantial savings from lower prescription costs," as the government would deal directly with drug makers. Furthermore, streamlined administration would save approximately $1.6 trillion. On the other side of the balance sheet, other provisions would drive up spending, including coverage for nearly thirty million uninsured, no deductibles and co-pays, and improved benefits, including dental, vision, and hearing.

Overall, while the study found that US health care spending under Sanders would drop over time, those potential savings would vanish, if hospitals and doctors are unwilling to accept lower fees for patients who are now privately insured. This gets us back to the lobbying power of the AMA and what it would be willing to accept on the part of its member base. Perhaps the most ambitious part of Sanders's Medicare for All is that it would do away with private health care insurance, by getting rid of "our complex, confusing, profit-driven mess of a health care system and start fresh with a single government-run insurer that would cover everyone" (Abelson and Sanger-Katz 2019). The issue here, however, is that it would also do away with an entire industry, one that employs at least half a million people, covers approximately 250 million Americans, and generates roughly a trillion dollars in revenues.

Additionally, private insurance stocks are an important part of mutual funds, which are part of retirement savings for millions of Americans. As such, the economic consequences of Sanders's Medicare for All haven't been analyzed thoroughly. The change would be hugely disruptive for the entire health care system, which makes up one-fifth of the US economy. Hospitals, doctors, nursing homes, and pharmaceutical companies would have to adapt to a new set of rules, while most Americans would have a new insurer: the federal government. As we've already noted, the federal government, and Congress, especially, hasn't done too well when it comes to covering health care for its veterans.

◆ Elizabeth Warren's Consumer Health Insurance Protection Act

Elizabeth Warren, the Democratic senator from Massachusetts, officially announced her bid for president in February 2019. However, unlike Sanders, her competitor, Warren is a fan of improving and strengthening the Affordable Care Act, rather than gutting it and putting in a universal health care focus. Her slogan, "affordable health care for every American," offers different ways to get there (Martin and Goodnough 2019).

One such way was a health care bill she introduced in March 2018, dubbed the Consumer Health Protection Act (Rosenberg 2018). This bill aimed to make insurance within the existing ACA more affordable, while protecting more enrollees from insurance company policy changes as well as premium hikes. Furthermore, the bill was geared toward increasing federal subsidies for those buying Affordable Care Act plans, while allowing more to qualify for additional ACA tax credits and imposing tighter controls on private insurers.

The Warren plan would also have

- offered limited insurance premiums to no more than 8.5 percent of income,

- capped out-of-pocket prescription drug costs for those on private plans at $250 a month (or $500 for families),
- required insurers who sell Medicare Advantage or Medicaid managed care plans to offer coverage on ACA exchanges with limited competition,
- required private insurance plans to spend 85 percent of the premiums received on paying out claims (under the ACA, the amount spent is 80 percent),
- provided more money for ACA outreach and enrollment efforts, and
- set limits on insurance company profits, to match what those private insurers can earn from Medicare and Medicaid

Co-sponsoring the bill were Sanders, along with Senators Kamala Harris (D-California), Maggie Hassan (D-New Hampshire), Kirsten Gillibrand (D-New York), and Tammy Baldwin (D-Wisconsin). While the bill didn't really go anywhere, it did indicate that "Democrats appear to be pulling together a plan that could win broad support within the party, and thus actually pass in some form if they retake Congress and the White House in 2020."

However, Warren, along with three other liberal presidential candidates (Harris, Gillibrand, and Cory Booker), did support a Medicare for All bill, which would create a government-run, single-payer health plan. But Warren, if not the others, seems to understand that Medicare for All is the long-term goal; at this time, short-term and significant plans would help "improve on the post-Donald Trump, post-Paul Ryan status quo," according to Bloomberg's Jonathan Bernstein.

◆ Kamala Harris: Get Rid of All Private Insurance

Senator Kamala Harris supports Sanders's Medicare for All and is backing Jayapal's bill. But Harris isn't interested in any kind of insurance for everyone or modified ACA. Rather, Harris indicated that things would be much better if private health insurance was completely abolished (Hains 2019). Such a move would go well beyond the single-payer systems in the United Kingdom and Canada. Both countries do have a private insurance industry to supplement the government-run health care systems.

Harris argues that under her system, patients would be liberated from patients going through third-party companies for approval, paperwork, and other delays that could get in the way of health care delivery. In a CNN town hall that took place in late January 2019, Harris advocated the elimination of what she dubbed the "inhumane" private health insurance industry. Also during that town hall meeting, she stressed that access to health care shouldn't be a privilege, which she believes it is now. Rather, health care should be understood to be a right. In terms of her feelings about the current state of affairs: "It's inhumane to make people go through a system where they cannot literally receive the benefit of what medical science can offer, because some insurance company has decided it doesn't meet their bottom line in terms of their profit motivation."

She is correct in that a true single-payer system would likely mean the end of private insurance. It would, instead, put everyone on a single, national health care plan. Here is the issue, however: In a poll conducted by the Kaiser Family Foundation, most Americans said they believed they would be able to keep their current insurance under a national health plan. However, that support dropped rapidly when they were told that the program would eliminate private insurance. Still, Harris's remarks are interesting, especially given that she has endorsed more incremental health care expansion plans that wouldn't do away 100 percent with insurance.

◆ Cory Booker: Against the High Cost of Drugs, But …

Finally, there is Senator Cory Booker (D-New Jersey); in January 2019, he appeared alongside Sanders at a press conference that involved lowering drug prices (Sullivan 2019). However, just two years earlier, Booker voted against a budget amendment that called for importing drugs from abroad. The reason for the flip-flop, and the somewhat soft response against higher drug prices, is because he receives contributions from the pharmaceutical industry. In 2014, he raised more money from the pharmaceutical industry than any other senator. New Jersey is home to the headquarters of many pharmaceutical companies. This eventually led Booker to announce he would refrain from taking contributions from drug companies. Still, he did end up drafting a revised importation bill that focused on better safety standards.

While he does seem to support Sanders and Medicare for All, many of the progressives are somewhat concerned that he is too deep in the pocket of corporate interests, especially the pharmaceutical industry. Furthermore, there is some concern that running against more progressive candidates, such as Warren and Sanders, could highlight perceptions that Booker doesn't stand up to corporate interests as best as he could.

However, one piece of sweeping legislation he mentioned in late January has raised the ire of Big Pharma (Sullivan 2019). The legislation would allow Medicare to negotiate drug prices, allow drugs to be imported from Canada, and strip monopolies from drug companies if their prices are higher than those in other wealthy countries. He has signed onto additional drug pricing as well, including a 2017 bill from former Sen. Al Franken (D-Minnesota), which would have allowed Medicare to negotiate drug prices. Booker also released a report in 2018 that criticized drug companies for not using savings from the Tax Cuts and Jobs Bill of 2017 to reduce drug prices.

There is little doubt that health care reform will be a top platform for many of the Democratic candidates as we move into the 2020 elections. As the primaries and speeches continue, there will, no doubt, be plenty of tweaking of the Medicare for All platform. However, the question is, even if a Democrat is elected to the presidency, will that individual have enough goodwill and support to actually overhaul a health care and insurance system that many Americans continue to like? Getting the Affordable Care Act passed has led to some stiff issues, as well as a political party that has tried to do its best to eliminate it. The Medicare Act created a great deal of animosity in the 1960s. And any time any president or Congress has attempted to push meaningful health care reform through as law, organizations and lobbyists amass and fight to keep things status quo.

CHAPTER NINE: FOCUS ON HEALTH CARE: THE PHYSICIAN SIDE

IN 2016, PHYSICIANS FOR A NATIONAL HEALTH PROGRAM (PNHP) released *Beyond the Affordable Care Act: A Physician's Proposal for Single-Payer Health Care Reform*. The gist of the plan pointed out the following:

- Even after full implementation of the ACA, tens of millions of Americans are either uninsured or partially insured.
- Health care costs are continuing to increase faster than the background inflation rate.
- The United States continues spending more on health care than other industrialized nations, while health care outcomes continue to lag behind, even with full ACA implementation.

"An estimated 27 million will remain uninsured, while many more face rising co-payments and deductibles that compromise access to care and leave them vulnerable to ruinous medical bills," the proposal noted (PNHP 2016). The working group that developed the proposal focused on the idea that a single-payer national health program, "an expansion of Medicare to the entire population," would cover all Americans for all needed medical care. The basics of the proposal are as follows.

◆ Coverage

When it comes to coverage, a single-payer NHP would cover every American citizen for all medically necessary services. This would include mental health, rehabilitation, and dental care, and coverage would be without co-payments or deductibles. Covered services would be determined by boards of experts and patient advocates, with ineffective services excluded from coverage.

◆ Hospitalization

In terms of hospital payments, the NHP would fund each hospital with a global budget, which consists of a lump sum that would cover all operating expenses. Doing so would eliminate per-patient billing, thus reducing administrative costs. Global budgets would be determined based on previous years' operating expenses, changes in demand and input prices, and proposed service enhancements. NHP would provide a separate, capital budget to fund expansion and modernization. "In Scotland and Canada, which fund hospitals through global budgets, administration consumes about 12% of hospital spending vs. 25% in the U.S.," the report said, adding that an NHP could shift about $150 billion annually from hospital administration to patient care.

◆ Physicians and Outpatient Care

An NHP would focus on two modes of payment for physicians and outpatient practitioners. The first, fee-for-service, would rely on a binding fee schedule. While the failings of health care tend to be blamed on fee-for-service incentives, the proposal notes that "other countries have found fee-for-service—as well as capitation and salaried practice—compatible with quality and cost containment." However, fees should not reward procedure-oriented specialists versus primary care physicians. The second is salaries for those working in nonprofit hospitals, HMOs, capitated group practices, and integrated health care systems. In these systems, hospitals and clinics could be paid through a separate global budget or a unified one for the entire organization.

◆ Long-Term Care

The proposal pointed out that Japan and Germany, which offer universal long-term care (LTC) coverage, provide more and better care, while not spending any more than what is spent in the United States. The long-term care program would also be covered under the NHP plan, with the organization funding a full spectrum of care for the disabled of all ages. Eligibility would be assessed by expert panels consisting of social workers, nurses, therapists, and physicians, with the agencies involved receiving a global budget. Under this plan, LTC would be provided in patients' homes and communities, rather than in institutions.

◆ Capital Investments and Improvements

The plan also takes into account capital investments for expansion and addition of new facilities and equipment, with the NHP funding these investments through specific appropriations. "When capital funding and operating payments are combined in a single revenue stream, as is now the case, profitable health care institutions are able to expand and modernize, regardless of medical needs, while those with less-favorable bottom lines fall behind," the report noted. The plan would avoid the current system, in which profits are made by avoiding unprofitable patients and services, as well as exercise of market clout.

◆ Training Programs

As a part of the planning process, the proposal suggests that training programs would produce an appropriate mix of health care professionals, while suggesting that residency programs train specialists and generalists in proportions that can meet societal needs. Part of the problem is that long-term debts incurred by medical students mean those students end up focused on higher-income specialties. To avoid this, the NHP would fully subsidize physician education, as well as the education of nurses, public health professionals, and other health care providers.

◆ Medications, Supplies, and Devices

In this particular area, the NHP would cover all medically necessary medications, devices, and supplies; to do this affordably, the NHP would directly negotiate prices with manufacturers. An expert panel would also be put in place to establish and update a national formulary which, in turn, would specify use of the lowest-cost medications among therapeutically equivalent drugs. The exception would be clinically required drugs. In addition, full drug coverage would be an essential component of an NHP; "co-payments reduce adherence to medications and worsen clinical outcomes," the report noted.

◆ Funding and Cost Containment

Finally, the single-payer system would "trim administration, reduce incentives to over-treat, lower drug prices, minimize wasteful investments in redundant facilities and eliminate almost all marketing and investor profits," the PNHP said. Total expenditures under the NHP would be limited to the same GDP proportion as the year prior to its establishment. During the transition period, all public funds spent on health care—which would include Medicare, Medicaid, and state and local health care programs—would be redirected to the NHO budget. While during the transition period, additional public funds could be raised by redirecting employers' health benefit spending through payroll taxes, the PNHP suggested that direct funding through progressive taxes over the long term would be fairer. "By unburdening employers, the NHP would facilitate entrepreneurship, while increasing the global competitiveness of American business," the report commented.

To conclude, while the PNHP has a good platform here, and one that makes a great deal of sense, the difficulty lies in passing any kind of meaningful health care reform. As mentioned throughout this book, it is highly difficult to come to a consensus on how it will happen.

CHAPTER TEN: THE ARGUMENT FOR MEDICARE FOR ALL

RESEARCH FROM BOTH SIDES OF THE SPECTRUM SHOW that Medicare for All, or at least a version of it, can achieve major cost savings in operations, relative to the current US health care system. "An Economic Analysis of Medicare for All," released by the Political Economic Research Institute at the University of Massachusetts/Amherst in late 2018, demonstrated that a Medicare for All type of program could reduce health care spending in the United States by nearly $2.93 trillion, below the $3.24 trillion it is currently at today (Pollin et al. 2018). Such a program would also help the 9 percent of US residents who have no insurance and the 26 percent who are underinsured; these are the people who are "unable to access needed care because of prohibitively high costs."

The authors of the study proposed that financing such a program would rely on the same revenue sources that provide about 60 percent of all US health care financing (such as Medicare and Medicaid), along with a 3.75 percent sales tax on nonnecessities and taxing long-term capital gains as ordinary income. Finally, a network tax of 0.38 percent could be placed on the first $1 million, which would apply to only the wealthiest 12 percent of US households.

The PERI study is not the only one indicating that the United States can afford true universal health care. When Charles Blahous at the Koch-funded Mercatus Center at George Mason University published a study suggesting that a single-payer health care plan would break the bank, observers pointed out that according to the Blahous estimates, a single-payer system would actually save Americans more than $2 trillion over a decade (Woolhandler, Himmelstein, and Gaffney 2018).

The reason why Blahous's estimates were incorrect was because single-payer will help promote administrative efficiency; billing costs primary care physicians $100,000 apiece while consuming 25 percent of emergency room revenues. Basically, close to one-third of all US health spending is due to bureaucracy. Noted Woolhandler et al., "Our profit-driven, multipayer system is the source for this outlandish administrative sprawl."

Meanwhile, even expanding health insurance coverage under the current ACA can help reduce health care costs. Economist Ray Perryman pointed out that his home state of Texas is one of fourteen that chose not to expand health insurance coverage to lower-income adults, using the Medicaid expansion coverage inherent in the Affordable Care Act. "Health care needs do not simply go away because individuals do not have insurance coverage," Perryman said (2019). In using Texas as an example, he noted that without health care coverage, medical issues escalate, leading to higher costs and worse outcomes (Perryman 2019). In fact, "Texas would gain over $110 billion in new federal health spending during the first 10 years."

His report went on to indicate notable improvements in states that have expanded coverage; in addition to improving health and well-being of those receiving coverage, the states experienced a reduction in the numbers of uninsured, as well as fewer emergency room visits. Other benefits have included improved health outcomes and enhanced employment and productivity.

In focusing on Texas, Perryman estimated that during the first ten years following an expansion implementation, net economic benefits would include $319.2 billion in real gross product, along with 3.3 million job-years in Texas (assuming use of multiplier effects). As such, for every dollar spent by the state of Texas for expanded insurance coverage, Perryman estimated that the total net economic spending would increase by $69.11, with real gross product increasing by $34.49 over the first ten years after implementation. Furthermore, estimated incremental tax receipts would include more than $19.5 billion to the state and more than $16.8 billion to local governments. In other words, while the state of Texas would be spending more on enhanced coverage, it would be receiving much more in return.

Perryman based his Texas study on the above-mentioned Kaiser Foundation study penned by Garfield et al. (2019). The researchers from that study noted that people in the coverage gap live below the poverty level, with limited family income; they are also likely employed in low-wage or part-time jobs or "with a fragile or unpredictable connection to the workforce." Furthermore, as many of these adults work in businesses that have little to no employer-based coverage, the analysts believe it's likely that they will continue to fall between the cracks of the employer-based system. And as mentioned above, people who fall into that coverage gap won't be able to afford coverage under the ACA, as they aren't eligible for the premium subsidies.

If these adults remain uninsured, as it seems as though they might, they are likely to continue facing barriers to health services and, when and if they do need medical care, could suffer potentially serious financial consequences. "Many are in fair or poor health, or are in the age range when health problems start to arise," Garfield et al. point out. However, because they don't have coverage, they are more likely to postpone needed care, due to the cost.

CHAPTER ELEVEN: CHALLENGES IN PASSING HEALTH CARE REFORM

WE ALREADY KNOW THAT THE CURRENT US HEALTH CARE system is simply unsustainable. It is too costly, too unwieldly, too confusing, and too cumbersome. We also know that switching to pure universal coverage (rather than the patchwork that is the Affordable Care Act) would likely alleviate many of the administrative costs burdening the health care system.

The major players in the US health services system include physicians, health service institution administrators, insurance companies, large employers, and the government (Shi et al. 1998). The negative effects of the often-conflicting self-interests of these players include the difficulty keeping tabs on myriad health plans; significant need for numerous claims processors; detail-oriented payment requirements that often result in denied claims, which in turn require more processing; issues with partial payment; lengthy collection efforts; and complex government programs. The positives are few and far between in a system that costs itself unnecessary expenses in exchange for comprehensive coverage for all.

Given the proof, through several studies, that either single-payer or a universal health care system would work, why is it so hard to get the concept moving in the United States? Why does any type of meaningful discussion about health care reform inevitably lead to hysteria or inaction? And why, above all, do legislators and politicians not even try to have an even-handed discussion about health care? Why do they insist on confusing the issue with bills that are nothing more than pages of legalese?

There are several reasons for this.

◆ US History

We pointed out earlier, US leaders have tried to reform health care as far back as before World War II. Going back even further, before World War I, some attempts were made to follow health care examples from Germany and others, for a universal health care system (Merelli 2017). These efforts were, however, met with opposition from doctors, insurance companies, businesses, and conservative labor organizations, "which considered state-sponsored health care paternalistic and unnecessary."

The labor unions, especially, were worried that state-sponsored health care might weaken their own bargaining power, as they felt they were responsible for obtaining social services for their members. That bias against state-sponsored insurance is alive and well today, as many Americans don't want government interfering with their health care coverage, even if that health care coverage isn't very good.

◆ Fear of Socialized Medicine

Political rhetoric and propaganda have always been used to fight comprehensive health care reform. The formalization of such rhetoric can be traced back to the 1940s and an organization called Campaigns Inc. Campaigns Inc. managed to quash any kind of government-sponsored health care plan by calling it "socialized medicine" and linking it to the Germans (in the early 1940s) and the Soviet Union (later on in the decade). These days, that socialistic fear remains, with many Americans convinced that universal health care coverage is a form of collectivism or socialism. The power of antisocialist rhetoric leads these Americans to believe that getting rid of the so-called free-market system we have today for one that is under control of the government will turn them into communists.

Furthermore, anything can be taken out of context. Remember the death panels that were going to be a hallmark of Obamacare, according to the bill's detractors? That whole concept came from something very innocent, namely, legislation allowing for end-of-life consultations to the terminally ill. That legislation was dropped, simply because it ended up being taken out of context and used to induce a type of hysteria. In an April 2017 survey conducted by YouGov, 60 percent of those queried answered positively to the idea of health care reform. Yet later on, in June 2017, when asked about introducing single-payer health care, only 44 percent asked agreed with the concept. As people continue to associate health care reform with socialized medicine, it will likely be difficult to pass any kind of meaningful health care reform.

◆ No Working-Class Representation

There are labor unions, of course. But there is no political party in the United States that specifically represents the working class, and without that labor party, social solidarity in issues such as health care is almost nonexistent. Though the Democratic Party does have ties with unions (including those who believe in European-style welfare policies), it also has ties to big business. This is the issue currently facing Sen. Corey Booker and his ties to Big Pharma; he is a Democrat dedicated to social welfare. Yet for a while, he accepted campaign contributions from the pharmaceutical industry.

Why has no true labor party emerged, even nonpolitically? Mainly because no large portion of US society believes it is truly "working class." Furthermore, the labor movement, in and of itself, is fragmented, especially when compared to other countries. For example, in some European countries, when one labor group strikes, others follow, in solidarity. This type of thing doesn't happen in the United States. Furthermore, those labor unions that do have some power in America tend to demonize anything that smacks of socialism.

◆ Powerful Lobbies

The medical and insurance lobbies are extremely powerful; we will take a closer look at the two main ones: the AMA and private insurance companies.

◆ The American Medical Association

The AMA was founded in 1847 with the goal of advancing the medical profession through better education at medical schools (AMA History). At the time, so-called "medical schools" were anything but, and the AMA focused on improving medical education and the quality of physicians graduating from those schools (AMA History).

These days, the AMA's mission is "to promote the science and art of medicine, and the betterment of public health" (American Medical Association 2019). On the positive side, the organization continues setting standards for medical schools and internship programs, while alerting the public to charlatans and quack medical remedies (American Medical Association 2019). However, the AMA is also a lobbying and advocacy group and has been the strongest opponent of a nationalized health care system.

This powerful physician group has regularly lobbied to prevent any kind of national comprehensive health care reform from passing, with the exception of the Affordable Care Act. In fact, the AMA's general opposition to Medicare and nationalized health insurance is due to the fact that it's not in the best interests of its membership. While the ACA, in theory, means more money for physicians (as it meant more patients would seek care), the more conservative members of the AMA tend to be disdainful of anything universal, for fear it might decrease doctors' wages (Meyer 2010). The individual mandate, according to Meyer in 2010, "reflects the physician organization's conflicted history with health care reform and universal coverage."

There could, however, be a chink in the AMA's armor, as younger members are increasingly coming out in support of universal health care (Luthra 2018). Specifically, the AMA's student caucus has, for years, been pushing for a resolution calling on the organization to drop its decades-long opposition to single-payer health care. During the annual meeting in summer 2018, the caucus finally got a hearing. While older physicians warned that under a universal system, doctor pay would decrease, by the end of the meeting, older members agreed to at least study the possibility of changing its position.

As older physicians retire and younger ones come up in the ranks, there could be a generational shift in the organization's stance. The "keep government out of my work" ethic, which characterized many physicians during the twentieth century, seems to be less of a factor among younger doctors. Furthermore, younger doctors, unlike their older counterparts, are more likely to end up working for large health systems or hospitals, as opposed to starting their own individual practices. Furthermore, young doctors seem to be more willing to explore what were considered previously unthinkable ideas. In a March 2018 *New England Journal of Medicine* survey, 61 percent of 607 respondents indicated that a single-payer system would make health care delivery more cost-effective. Still, doctors represent only one part of the health care industrial complex.

◆ Private Insurance Companies

There is no doubt that private insurance companies are probably the largest obstacle to any kind of meaningful health care reform, whether that reform encompasses a single-payer system or full insurance coverage. As of this writing, insurance lobbyists have been marshalling financial and other resources to fight against universal coverage, and for good reason (Stein 2019). Basically, a Medicare for All plan would legislate many private insurance companies out of existence.

In one meeting with employees, United Healthcare chief executive Steve Nelson indicated that the company opposes Medicare for All, as it excludes the private sector (Stein 2019). And the private sector does a better job of health care delivery than the government, Nelson said. However, the main fight against universal coverage, from the private insurance side, is that of profit loss. "These companies completely understand that the federal government can discipline prices, and that doing so could have a fundamental impact on every single thing in their business," according to University of Chicago health care expert Harold Pollack.

The final issue, which really can't be ignored, is that the private insurance industry, especially as it focuses on health care, is a huge part of the economy. Health care, as a whole, represents one-sixth of the US GDP; a radical change on the private insurance end could have far-reaching economic consequences. Profit motive aside, insurance companies do have cause for concern with any kind of health care change. It was, in fact, the private insurance companies that lobbied against the single-payer option in the ACA; that option was eventually dropped from the final legislation.

Over the past century, both the AMA and private insurance lobbyists have done a very good job of opposing nonprofit and universal health care, understanding it would mean less in their particular coffers. As such, any kind of legislation involving health care reform runs against the resources and brick wall of lobbyists determined to make the current system remain in place. For example, the health care and insurance lobbies are already rallying around to kill the Medicare for All plan. "Doctors, hospitals, drug companies and insurers are intent on strangling Medicare for all before it advances from an aspirational slogan to a legislative agenda item," Robert Pear wrote in the *New York Times* (February 2019).

The groups have banded together into one coalition, Partnership for America's Health Care Future, to create and deliver digital advertising, videos, and Twitter posts, in an attempt to reach hearts and minds when it comes to this topic (Pear 2019). The coalition includes the American Medical Association, the American Hospital Association, and the nation's Blue Cross and Blue Shield plans. As noted above, slogans and assumptions have had a powerful influence on public opinion, causing it to sway against issues such as Medicare for All or any other meaningful change.

Nor is this the only time during which Big Pharma, the AMA, and other powerful lobbies have banded together to defeat universal health care. As indicated earlier, repeated attempts by presidents and Congress to pass meaningful health care reform have been stymied, meaning the bills die in committee before they can make it to the voting floor. With such a dismal past record, it's difficult to determine why this time would be much different, no matter who is in the White House or Congress.

◆ Racial Undercurrents

This interesting factor isn't typically mentioned. However, Shen and LaBouff, in a study, focused on the idea that racism could also be a reason why a single-payer system or universal health care might be hard to swallow. The researchers pointed out that first of all, race ended up being a salient influence on political attitudes when Barack Obama, the nation's first black president, took office. Because Obama was the author of the ACA, attitudes toward him also spilled over toward attitudes toward his policies. In conducting a specific study among participants concerning subtle racism and government aid programs (such as health care), the researchers noted a "correlational relationship between subtle racial prejudice and opposition to universal healthcare" but acknowledged that the causal links weren't as clear.

Still, the race of individuals seeking universal health care also influenced the degree of acceptance; basically, when it was suggested that recipients of universal health care might be black, survey participants were less likely to accept it. Isn't there racism in other countries? There is. But one thing we need to remember is that other countries have had some form of single-payer or universal health care present, whereas this has been a stumbling block in the United States. While racism isn't the sole reason for the anti-universal health care sentiment, it could play somewhat of a role in a country that was not 100 percent behind its black president.

◆ Another Issue: How Would It Work?

The question to answer here is whether a mixed system (similar to Canada) or a 100 percent government-sponsored system (such as in the United Kingdom) could be effective in the United States. Needless to say, over the years, experts have weighed pros and cons when it comes to a national health insurance program. Mark Pauley, professor of health care management and business economics and public policy at the University of Pennsylvania's Wharton School of Business, indicated that "the question is whether it will work better than either what we currently have, which is not a very high bar, or whether it will work better than some other alternatives" (Pauley and Field 2019). He went on to suggest that a single-payer plan would increase the tax burden, while raising questions such as, should all care be free for everyone? Who decides how that care will be paid for? And furthermore, should insurance be socialized or should private firms have a role in this scenario?

Another question that Pauley brings up is that if the government has to pay its share in a Medicare for All type of plan, one way to finance it would be to double the income tax for everyone who pays for it. However, if the higher taxes replace employer-provided health insurance, employees might expect higher wages. The other question revolves around overuse of the system; if out-of-pocket costs (such as co-pays and deductibles) are removed, does this mean that people might overuse medical services? Other questions concerning a universal health care system focus on how care can be delivered economically (Pauley and Field 2019).

In short, simply abolishing private insurance companies would lead to a host of other questions. There is the problem of literally upending one-sixth of the US economy, the one that employs and pays health care and insurance workers. Furthermore, while a consensus has, at least on the Democratic side, developed using Medicare for a single-payer health care system, Medicare isn't a single-payer system (Holland 2017). It is, in fact, a government-sponsored program for basics in care (that enrollees need to pay for), combined with private plans purchased under the Medicare Advantage program.

According to Joshua Holland, approximately one-third of Medicare enrollees purchased a private plan under this program; they have increased in popularity, mainly because the field has been tilted against the traditional, government-run program. For example, Medicare Advantage plans require a cap on out-of-pocket costs, but the public program doesn't. Approximately one in four Medicare enrollees purchased the Medigap policy to cover out-of-pocket costs (Holland 2017). Furthermore, there are public and private prescription drug plans (Holland 2017). The confusion led Holland to note that Medicare, as it currently stands, is "a far cry from the simplicity that single-payer systems promise."

Holland also points out that while Medicare for All seems to be an attractive slogan, it isn't a good tool to get from where we are now, with the current health care system, to where we need to be. Even the experts touting Medicare for All proposals note that the ones currently on the table are likely to be highly difficult to enact. For one thing, they aren't likely to include enough time to transition from the current health care system to a different one. The ACA was passed in 2010 and was implemented in 2013, and the initial implementation was a mess, between confusion over health care exchanges and crashing websites. Two years is simply not long enough.

Sanders's most recent bill, for example, doesn't propose a timeline, but his 2013 American Health Security Act indicated a two-year transition period. "Radically restructuring a sixth of the economy in such short order would be like trying to stop a cruise ship on a dime," Holland pointed out. For one thing, forcing the entire population to move to a Medicare-for-All program, especially over a short period of time, will likely lead to a massive backlash, a concept known as "loss aversion." People tend to value something they already have far more than what they might value if they were forced to give something up. This is one reason why the Democrats faced such problems after the ACA was passed and why Republicans, less than a decade later, prevented the ACA rollback.

President Barack Obama faced a huge firestorm when his promise that people could keep their insurance backfired after 1.6 million people lost their substandard plans under the act (Holland 2017). While the ACA did extend coverage to almost ten times as many people (and, in many cases, under better plans), those who lost their insurance caused the right to rally around the law, a fight that is still going on today.

Basically, while there are several policies on the table touting a single-payer system, Harold Pollack, University of Chicago public-health researcher and liberal advocate for universal coverage, has pointed out the problem of a detailed single-payer bill that lays out transitional issues. "Even if you believe everything people say about the cost savings that would result," Pollack added, "there are still so many detailed questions about how we should finance this, how we can deal with the shock to the system, and so on."

Under current Medicare for All proposals, more than 70 percent of the adult population would be forced into such a program, and this would include tens of millions of people who currently have decent coverage from employers, the VHA, and the Federal Employees Health Benefits Program. In fact, many employer-provided policies cover more than Medicare does, meaning a "for-all" expansion could mean lots of people might objectively lose out in the deal. A single-payer system would be asking one-third of seniors to give up their heavily subsidized Medicare Advantage plans. Furthermore, as some doctors could decline to participate in a single-payer situation, it's possible that people might not be able to keep their physicians under such a plan.

Holland's contention wasn't that a single-payer plan might not work but, rather, that forcing a lot of people to move into a new system "is all but guaranteed to result in tons of resistance." And that is without taking into account attacks from conservatives, the same group that converted some funds for voluntary end-of-life counseling into "death panels." Holland also blasted the common perception that because single-payer systems in other parts of the world cost so much less than ours, passage of a single-payer mandate would bring spending in line with what the rest of the world pays.

While there could be some savings on administrative costs, the rest of the world established their systems when they weren't spending a lot on health care and were able to keep prices down through aggressive cost controls. Even with this, most countries with single-payer systems rely on some combination of public insurance, mixes of mandatory and voluntarily private insurance (typically tightly regulated), and out-of-pocket expenditures that are capped. Basically, the United States isn't unique in mixing public and private financing; the difference is that Americans rely more heavily on private insurance than do other wealthy countries.

Then there are the American people, themselves. The United States has what Hacker calls a "fragmented and exorbitantly expensive system." But that system also all but guarantees that every reasonably well-insured group (whether employees through employer-sponsored health care plans or Medicare beneficiaries) will automatically be distrustful of change as well as sensitive to new costs, even if those costs replace the hidden charges they are paying. More than 150 million Americans are covered by employment-based health plans; even as these plans are becoming less common, more expensive, and more restrictive, this is half of the US population. Those with workplace coverage are generally satisfied with that coverage, with Medicare beneficiaries even happier.

Finally, financing a huge transition to single-payer would be a large challenge. Most well-insured Americans have no idea how much they are actually paying; what they see is a portion of the premium and out-of-pocket spending (Hacker 2018). What they are actually paying is greater and includes lower wages they receive because they receive health benefits instead of cash. It also encompasses higher taxes paid on everything else; the government receives lower revenues because it doesn't tax medical benefits as pay. Noted Hacker, "Our system is almost perfectly designed to hide the true costs of health care." This is because those who benefit from a lack of transparency (drug companies, highly paid specialists, medical device manufacturers, and commercial insurance companies) want it that way.

The system also enriches stakeholders who are willing to spend whatever it takes to block changes that threaten them. Basically, any plan liability will be located and then exploited. For example, when President Clinton described his health care plan before a joint session of Congress, it garnered majority support among voters.

Following a few months of GOP and industry attacks, the poll numbers dropped.

Medicare for All would bring those costs into the open, but those with good coverage would suddenly face a steep tax bill for something they believe they were getting inexpensively.

CHAPTER TWELVE: UNIVERSAL HEALTH CARE? OR BETTER HEALTH CARE?

WHILE THE UNITED STATES WRESTLES WITH THE IDEA OF Medicare for All and wonders how the heck to contain increasingly out-of-control health care costs, it bears reminding that just because everyone has access to insurance to pay for health care doesn't mean that they have access to it. Many times, having the right insurance, or not having to pay for health care, doesn't mean that everyone will have access to it. As such, perhaps the problem isn't not enough health insurance. Perhaps the basic problem with the US health care system is that too much is being spent on health care, with far too little received in return for the health care dollar (US PIRG 2018). Furthermore, excessive costs can be attributed to waste, which doesn't actually improve quality of care.

One good example of this is the patient who is under the care of a cardiologist, nephrologist, and infectious disease doctor, with all three requiring three separate blood tests, when one could have done the trick. There is no one entity that is coordinating the care, that is taking responsibility for the blood draw and making sure it is available to these specialists. So while the United States wrestles with getting some kind of Medicare for All bill through legislation and the inevitable backlash, the United States Public Interest Research Group issued suggestions on how to make health care work better, in other words, make it more cost-effective, with better outcomes. For example, get the basics right. While America's health care system is known for developing advanced treatments, many times, it fails to provide effective low-cost treatments that would work, triggering unnecessary treatments and higher cost down the road. Here are some of their other suggestions:

◆ Invest in Prevention

The current health care system rewards hospitals and doctors for performing as many procedures as possible, without much consideration as to whether they keep people out of the hospital. More effort should be put toward preventative services.

◆ Increase Safe Health Care

Experts suggest that medical errors are the third most common cause of death in the United States, but little is being done to reduce those statistics.

◆ Hold Insurers Accountable

Health insurance rate hikes receive little scrutiny. As mentioned already, private insurance companies have no incentives to be transparent with rate hikes or other information. Furthermore, there isn't much oversight to ensure that insurance companies are delivering on their commitments to members. Focusing on insurers' payment strategies, along with quantitative goals and results, can help other efforts to improve safety, increase care coordination and prevention, and bring down health care costs for consumers.

◆ Prescription Drug Reform

Drug development and the patent system means higher prices for developing and marketing the next blockbuster drug, rather than focusing on needed therapies for life-threatening conditions. Overhauling the patent system will reduce the pricing power of pharmaceutical companies.

◆ Make Prices Available to Consumers

People should get prices for services and treatments up front, so they can make informed decisions about value and encourage price competition to help keep costs in check. Get rid of the charge master, that huge document, and instead, focus on simple listing of prices.

◆ Public Option Health Plan

This allows Americans under the age of sixty-five to buy into Medicare or Medicaid, which could in turn provide a cheaper alternative to commercial health insurance.

◆ Shift the Payment Model

One problem with the traditional fee-for-service plan is that it focuses on individual services and volume, as opposed to quality or positive results. During the past several decades, little has been done to discourage this way of doing business or to motivate health care providers to collaborate, so as to figure out the most cost-effective course of treatments that will yield the best patient outcomes.

◆ Do a Better Job with Data

A great deal of data exists in the health care field. That is the good news. The not-so-good news is that even with all the available data, actual costs and outcome numbers aren't available, not to payers, not to consumers, and not even to the doctors or other health care providers. This aligns with Brill's description of the charge master, which can vary, not just from service to service, but from hospital to hospital. Basically, without an understanding of actual costs and outcomes, any goal involving cutting waste and boosting efficiency isn't going to be very effective. The $3 trillion annual price tag for US health care reflects the amount that providers charge, not the actual cost of care (Martinez, King, and Cauchi 2016).

Even more disturbing to contemplate is that a study on this issue, reported in the *Harvard Business Review*, noted that few hospitals or health care organizations have accurate information on actual costs (Porter and Lee 2013).

◆ Organize into Integrated Practice Units

This proposal takes the concept of the ACO one step further, by organizing health care delivery around a patient's medical condition (Porter and Lee 2013). It involves treating not only a disease but related conditions and circumstances that can sometimes occur with it (Porter and Lee 2013). A patient who is diagnosed with diabetes, for example, would also have immediate access to a nephrologist (for potential kidney disorders) and an ophthalmologist (for eye checkups), without having to deal with the time and trouble of looking up yet another specialist and waiting for an appointment.

This concept is especially important when it comes to the sickest and most frail patients in the US health care system; this is the group that generally requires the most intense and expensive medical care. Basically, the top 5 percent of patients, ranked by health care expenditures, accounted for half of the nation's health care expenditures, due to the complexity of their illnesses or conditions. Furthermore, the Commonwealth Fund found out that 24 percent of US primary care doctors indicated that their practices aren't prepared to manage care for patients with multiple chronic diseases. Additionally, 84 percent of those surveyed indicated that they aren't prepared for patients with severe mental illnesses who, along with patients who have chronic illnesses, tend to be among the sickest patients.

CHAPTER THIRTEEN: THOUGHTS FOR REFORM

BACK IN 2009, MANCHIKANTI AND HIRSH POINTED OUT that the interests of those involved in health care are divergent and often don't represent the importance of the need of health care for vulnerable populations. This is as true today as it was in 2009, when President Obama was attempting to negotiate and push through health care reform.

Health care reform impacts different groups in different ways, from physicians and providers to employers, insurers, and even politicians and advocacy groups. And yes, some of these groups are going to be negatively impacted by the transition towards any kind of national health care service or nationalized insurance program. We've focused on the many reasons why meaningful health care reform, either universal coverage or single-payer, will be difficult to implement. It will be difficult but not impossible. One of the misnomers, though, is that the existence of divergent interests means that a program cannot be developed. Smaller strides have been made in some areas. And on a large-scale effort, the UK demonstrated that efforts can be made towards changes that involve large-scale programming alterations and that successful outcomes can be achieved.

In 2008, the United Kingdom introduced new requirements for primary care office practices; over a forty-four-month period, it transformed the fifty-five hundred primary care offices serving thirty-two million individuals towards a prevention strategy in relation to coronary artery disease. Certainly, the transformation took time and did lead to frustration and anger. However, there was the belief that collaborative activities can be achieved, and improvements implemented across industries are clearly identifiable in relation to the health care process.

Basically, our legislators and lobbyists need to stop treating health care like a weapon to hit each other over the head with and focus on better ways to bring national interests together. President Obama was able to do this with the Affordable Care Act, and while that legislation passed along party lines, it did secure the support of many of the stakeholders involved.

Regardless of whatever health care reform is passed, the following should be the goals of any program:

- to provide health care
- to completely reform the health care system and end incentives for costly expenditures
- to reform the market-based insurance system and push insurers to pursue high-end insurance options for noncovered conditions
- to reduce administrative waste
- to align patient needs with the activities of health care organizations and providers

Some of the elements of the physician plans that have been introduced are valuable when considering an overall effort to meet the needs of the country as a whole. These elements include inclusion provisions; the focus on multiple funding mechanisms on the state and federal level; the use of employer taxation that would meet current levels of health insurance payments; the stipulations regarding administrative process and reimbursement procedures; and the use of technology for the standardization of reporting measures. In addition, methods should be included in the plan for supporting fraud prevention activities in alignment with regulations currently in place under Medicare and Medicaid.

A decade ago, Robert Yates stated that the World Health Organization had recognized the need for improvements in health care coverage and implored countries to implement universal coverage for all citizens as a part of their Millennium Development Goals. In fact, the WHO international panel maintained the importance of improving health outcomes as a component of addressing international poverty but also identified the current health care scenarios in countries like the United States as problematic in relation to poverty. Specifically, WHO has maintained that taking money from poor people who are sick is never a good idea and that reductions in poverty and improvements in health are linked to the need for an improved health care system in this country.

Proposals have reflected the importance of balancing the needs of the most vulnerable populations with an administrative process that places control in the hands of state governments to allocate resources and determine methods for implementing a national health strategy. One of the most difficult components of this process is that large insurers and pharmaceutical companies have invested significantly in the current free-market system and so will utilize their resources to fight against measures to replace their functions in the industry. They are already doing so during the run-up to the 2020 presidential election and will likely continue, no matter who ends up winning the White House.

Though this kind of transformation may appear daunting, many countries have implemented national health programs with an existing infrastructure in place and have been successful at achieving improvements in health care access across populations.

REFERENCES

Abelson, R., and M. Sanger-Katz. March 23, 2019. "Medicare for All Would Abolish Private Insurance." Retrieved from *New York Times*: https://www.nytimes.com/2019/03/23/health/private-health-insurance-medicare-for-all-bernie-sanders.html

Alonso-Zaldivar, R. July 30, 2018. "Study: 'Medicare for All' Projected to Cost $36.2 Trillion." Retrieved from Associated Press: https://www.apnews.com/09e06d686a1a481fa76e3fd91f3fcbc2

Altman, S. H. September 2012. "The Lessons of Medicare's Prospective Payment System Show that the Bundled Payment Program Faces Challenges." Retrieved from Health Affairs: https://www.healthaffairs.org/doi/full/10.1377/hlthaff.2012.0323

AMA History. (n.d.) Retrieved from https://www.ama-assn.org/about/ama-history/ama-history

American Medical Association. 2009. "Health Systems Reform: Legislative Summary Chart of Major Provisions." Retrieved from http://www.ama-assn.org/ama1/pub/upload/mm/399/hsr-hr3962-hr3590-comparison-chart.pdf

American Medical Association. May 3, 2019. Retrieved from Encyclopedia Britannica: https://www.britannica.com/topic/American-Medical-Association

Bartlett, D. L., and J. B. Steele. 2004. *Critical Condition: How Health Care in America Became Big Business and Bad Medicine*. New York: Doubleday.

Belluz, J. April 8, 2019. "The Absurdly High Cost of Insulin, Explained." Retrieved from Vox: https://www.vox.com/2019/4/3/18293950/why-is-insulin-so-expensive

Bendavid, N. July 18, 2017. "Why Obamacare Passed but the GOP Health Bill Failed." Retrieved from *Wall Street Journal*: https://www.commonwealthfund.org/sites/default/files/documents/____media_files_publications_issue_brief_2016_sep_1903_saltzman_trump_hlt_care_reform_proposals_ib_v2.pdf

Blue Cross and Blue Shield Association History. 2014. International Directory of Company Histories, Vol 10. Boston: St. James Press (Cengage). Retrieved from Funding Universe: http://www.fundinguniverse.com/company-histories/blue-cross-and-blue-shield-association-history/

Blumenthal, D. December 5, 2017. "The Decline of Employer-Sponsored Health Insurance." Retrieved from the Commonwealth Fund: https://www.commonwealthfund.org/blog/2017/decline-employer-sponsored-health-insurance

Brill, Steven. March 4, 2013. "Bitter Pill. Why Medical Bills Are Killing Us." *Time* Magazine. Retrieved from http://content.time.com/time/subscriber/article/0,33009,2136864,00.html

Brodie, M., E. C. Hamel, and M. Norton. 2015. "Medicare as Reflected in Public Opinion." Retrieved from American Society on Aging: https://www.asaging.org/blog/medicare-reflected-public-opinion

Carroll, A. E. September 5, 2017. "The Real Reason the U.S. Has Employer-Sponsored Health Insurance." Retrieved from *New York Times*: https://www.nytimes.com/2017/09/05/upshot/the-real-reason-the-us-has-employer-sponsored-health-insurance.html

Cherelus, G. January 8, 2019. "New York City Launches $100 Million Universal Health Insurance Program." Retrieved from Reuters: https://www.reuters.com/article/us-new-york-healthcare/new-york-city-launches-100-million-universal-health-insurance-program-idUSKCN1P21WF

Clymer, A., R. Pear, and R. Toner. August 29, 1994. "The Healthcare Debate: What Went Wrong?" Retrieved from *New York Times*: https://www.nytimes.com/1994/08/29/us/health-care-debate-what-went-wrong-health-care-campaign-collapsed-special-report.html

Courtemanche, C., J. Marton, B. Ukert, A. Yelowitz, and D. Zapata. August 2018. "Effects of the Affordable Care Act on Health Care Access and Self-Assessed Health after 3 Years." Retrieved from *INQUIRY: The Journal of Health Care Organization, Provision and Financing*: https://journals.sagepub.com/doi/full/10.1177/0046958018796361

Dorn, S. D. December 2017. "Repeal and Replace? Repair or Despair? 2017 Health Care Reform and Clinical Gastroenterology." *Gastroenterology*, 153(6), 1465–1468.

Dropp, K., and B. Nyhan. February 7, 2017. "One-Third Don't Know Obamacare and Affordable Care Act Are the Same." Retrieved from *New York Times*: https://www.nytimes.com/2017/02/07/upshot/one-third-dont-know-obamacare-and-affordable-care-act-are-the-same.html

Facts & Data on Small Business and Entrepreneurship. 2017. Small Business & Entrepreneurship Council. Retrieved from https://sbecouncil.org/about-us/facts-and-data/

Frakt, A. May 14, 2018. "Medical Mystery: Something Happened to U.S. Health Spending after 1980." Retrieved from *New York Times*: https://www.nytimes.com/2018/05/14/upshot/medical-mystery-health-spending-1980.html

Frakt, A. June 4, 2018. "Reagan, Deregulation and America's Exceptional Rise in Health Care Costs." Retrieved from *New York Times*: https://www.nytimes.com/2018/06/04/upshot/reagan-deregulation-and-americas-exceptional-rise-in-health-care-costs.html

Frayer, L. March 7, 2018. "U.K. Hospitals Are Overburdened, but the British Love Their Universal Health Care." Retrieved from NPR: https://www.npr.org/sections/parallels/2018/03/07/591128836/u-k-hospitals-are-overburdened-but-the-british-love-their-universal-health-care

Freeman, G. A. December 20, 2017. "Health Plans Leave Middle Class with Few Options." Retrieved from Health Leaders: https://www.healthleadersmedia.com/finance/health-plans-leave-middle-class-few-options

Garfield, R., K. Orgera, and A. Damico. March 21, 2019. "The Coverage Gap: Uninsured Poor Adults in States that Do

Not Expand Medicaid." Retrieved from Kaiser Permanente Foundation: https://www.kff.org/medicaid/issue-brief/the-coverage-gap-uninsured-poor-adults-in-states-that-do-not-expand-medicaid/

Gersema, E. April 5, 2018. "High-Deductible Health Plans Raise Risk of Financial Ruin for Vulnerable Americans, Study Finds." Retrieved from *USC News*: https://news.usc.edu/140182/high-deductible-health-plans-raise-risk-of-financial-ruin-for-vulnerable-americans-study-finds/

Gold, J. September 14, 2015. "Accountable Care Organizations, Explained." Retrieved from *Kaiser Health News*: https://khn.org/news/aco-accountable-care-organization-faq/

Griffin, J. March 7, 2017. "The History of Healthcare in America." Retrieved from J. P. Griffin Group: https://www.griffinbenefits.com/employeebenefitsblog/history_of_healthcare

Hacker, J. S. January 3, 2018. "The Road to Medicare for Everyone." Retrieved from *American Prospect*: https://prospect.org/article/road-medicare-everyone

Hains, T. January 29, 2019. "Kamala Harris on Private Health Insurance Market: 'Eliminate That,' 'Let's Move On.'" Retrieved from Real Clear Politics: https://www.realclearpolitics.com/video/2019/01/29/kamala_harris_on_private_health_insurance_market_eliminate_all_of_that_lets_move_on.html

Hansler, Jennifer. September 13, 2017. "A Short American History: From Medicare to Obamacare to ... Berniecare?" CNN. Retrieved from https://www.cnn.com/2017/09/13/politics/history-of-us-health-care/index.html.

Haseltine, W. A. April 2, 2018. "Aging Populations Will Challenge Healthcare Systems All over the World." Retrieved from *Forbes*: https://www.forbes.com/sites/williamhaseltine/2018/04/02/aging-populations-will-challenge-healthcare-systems-all-over-the-world/#7cca91942cc3

Hirsch, J. A., A. B. Rosenkrantz, G. N. Nicola, H. B. Harvey, R. Duszak Jr., E. Silva III, L. Manchikanti, et al. 2017. "Contextualizing the First-Round Failure of the AHCA: Down but Not Out." *Journal of NeuroInterventional Surgery* 9, 595–600. doi:10.1136/neurintsurg-2017-013136

Holland, J. August 2, 2017. "Medicare-for-All Isn't the Solution for Universal Health Care." Retrieved from *The Nation*: https://www.thenation.com/article/medicare-for-all-isnt-the-solution-for-universal-health-care/

How Much. 2018. "Here Are the Most and Least Expensive States for Health Insurance." Retrieved from https://howmuch.net/articles/health-insurance-rates-by-state

"Introduction to Medicare." 2019. Retrieved from Medicare Interactive: https://www.medicareinteractive.org/get-answers/medicare-basics/medicare-overview/introduction-to-medicare

Khullar, D., and D. A. Chokshi. October 4, 2018. "Health, Income & Poverty: Where We Are & What Could Help." Retrieved from Health Affairs: https://www.healthaffairs.org/do/10.1377/hpb20180817.901935/full/

Lee, T. H. and K. Zapert. September 22, 2005. "Do High-Deductible Health Plans Threaten Quality of Care?" *New England Journal of Medicine* 353, 1202-1204. DOI: 10.1056/NEJMp058209

Levy, M. March 16, 2019. "Patient Protection and Affordable Care Act." Retrieved from Encyclopaedia Britannica: https://www.britannica.com/topic/Patient-Protection-and-Affordable-Care-Act

Long, S. K., and J. Aaron. December 2018. "Near-Universal Health Insurance Coverage in Massachusetts: Gaps in Health Care Access and Affordability Persisted into 2018." Retrieved from Blue Cross Foundation Massachusetts: https://bluecrossmafoundation.org/sites/default/files/2018_MHRS%20Chartpack%20CORE%20Measures_final.pdf

Long, S. K., L. Skopec, A. Shelto, K. Nordahl, and K. K. Walsh. 2016. "Massachusetts Health Reform at Ten Years: Great Progress, but Coverage Gaps Remain." *Health Affairs* 35(9), 1633–37. doi:10.1377/hlthaff.2016.0354

Longman, P. April 14, 2018. "Five Myths about the Veterans Affairs Health Care." Retrieved from *Newsday*: https://www.newsday.com/opinion/commentary/5-myths-about-the-veterans-affairs-health-care-1.18016058

Luthra, S. August 1, 2018. "The Next Generation of Doctors Is Pushing for Universal Healthcare." Retrieved from *Tonic/Kaiser Health News*: https://tonic.vice.com/en_us/article/43p44n/american-medical-association-single-payer-universal-healthcare

Manchikanti, L., and J. Hirsch. 2009. "Health Policy: Obama Care for All Americans: Practical Implications." *Pain Physician* 12, 289–304. Retrieved from http://www.painphysicianjournal.com/2009/march/2009;12;289-304.pdf

Manchikanti, L., S. Helm II, R. M. Benyamin, and J. A. Hirsch. March 2017. "Evolution of U.S. Health Care Reform." *Pain Physician* 20(3), 107–110.

Martin, J., and A. Goodnough. February 2, 2019. "Medicare for All Emerges as Early Policy Test for 2020 Democrats." Retrieved from *New York Times*: https://www.nytimes.com/2019/02/02/us/politics/medicare-for-all-2020.html

Martinez, J. C., M. P. King, and R. Cauchi. 2016. "Improving the Health Care System: Seven State Strategies." National Conference of State Legislators.

Mechanic, D. 2004. "The Rise and Fall of Managed Care." *Journal of Health and Social Behavior* 45, 76–86.

Meinert, M. June 21, 2018. "Seniors Will Soon Outnumber Children, but the U.S. Isn't Ready." Retrieved from *USC News*: https://news.usc.edu/143675/aging-u-s-population-unique-health-challenges/

Merelli, A. July 18, 2017. "A History of Why the U.S. Is the Only Rich Country without Universal Health Care." Retrieved from Quartz: https://qz.com/1022831/why-doesnt-the-united-states-have-universal-health-care/

Meyer, Harris. November 3, 2010. "AMA Conservatives Revolt against the Individual Mandate." Retrieved from Health Affairs: https://www.healthaffairs.org/do/10.1377/hblog20101130.008103/full/

Montgomery, K. March 20, 2019. "Differences between Universal Coverage and Single-Payer." Retrieved from Very Well Health: https://www.verywellhealth.com/difference-between-universal-coverage-and-single-payer-system-1738546

Morgan, R., and H. Nicholson. June 23, 2017. "Overview: Better Care Reconciliation Act of 2017." Retrieved from National Conference of State Legislatures: http://www.ncsl.org/research/health/overview-better-care-reconciliation-act-of-2017.aspx

Moseley III, George B. 2008. "The U.S. Health Care Non-System, 1908–2008." Retrieved from *AMA Journal of Ethics*: https://journalofethics.ama-assn.org/article/us-health-care-non-system-1908-2008/2008-05

Nash, D. September 21, 2018. "Are Accountable Care Organizations Saving Money, or Not?" Retrieved from *MedPage Today*: https://www.medpagetoday.com/columns/focusonpolicy/75239

National Health Expenditure Data—Historical. December 2018. Retrieved from Centers for Medicare & Medicaid Services: https://www.cms.gov/research-statistics-data-and-systems/statistics-trends-and-reports/nationalhealthexpenddata/nationalhealthaccountshistorical.html

Newkirk, V. R. March 4, 2016. "Medicare Is Leaving Elderly Women Behind." Retrieved from *The Atlantic*: https://www.theatlantic.com/politics/archive/2016/03/elderly-women-medicare-issues/472155/

NPR. 2015. "'America's Bitter Pill' Makes Case for 'Why Health Care Law Won't Work.'" Retrieved from National Public Radio: https://www.npr.org/sections/health-shots/2015/01/05/375024427/americas-bitter-pill-makes-case-for-why-health-care-law-wont-work

OECD. 2017. "Health at a Glance 2017: OECD Indicators." Paris: OECD Publishing. doi:https://dx.doi.org/10.1787/health_glance-2017-en

O'Neill, J. E., and D. M. O'Neill. September 2007. "Health Status, Health Care and Inequality: Canada vs. the U.S." Cambridge, MA: National Bureau of Economic Research. doi:https://www.nber.org/papers/w13429.pdf

O'Shea, J. June 24, 2016. "Reforming Veterans Health Care: Now and for the Future." Retrieved from the Heritage Foundation: https://www.heritage.org/health-care-reform/report/reforming-veterans-health-care-now-and-the-future

Papanicolas, I., L. R. Woskie, and A. K. Jha. March 13, 2018. "Healthcare Spending in the United States and Other High-Income Countries." Retrieved from *JAMA Network*: https://jamanetwork.com/journals/jama/article-abstract/2674671

Pauley, M., and R. Field. February 22, 2019. "Could Universal Health Care Work in the U.S.?" Retrieved from Wharton, the University of Pennsylvania: http://knowledge.wharton.upenn.edu/article/could-universal-health-care-work-in-the-u-s/

Pear, R. February 23, 2019. "Health Care and Insurance Industries Mobilize to Kill 'Medicare for All.'" Retrieved from *New York Times*: https://www.nytimes.com/2019/02/23/us/politics/medicare-for-all-lobbyists.html

Perryman, R. March 28, 2019. "Economic Benefits of Expanding Health Insurance Coverage in Texas." Retrieved from the Perryman Group: https://www.perrymangroup.com/economic-benefits-of-expanding-health-insurance-coverage-in-texas/

PNHP. 2016. "Beyond the Affordable Care Act: A Physician's Proposal for Single-Payer Health Care Reform." Retrieved from Physicians for a National Health Plan: https://pnhp.org/beyond_aca/Physicians_Proposal.pdf

Pollack, Andrew September 20, 2015. "Drug Goes from $13.50 a Tablet to $750, Overnight." Retrieved from *New York Times*: https://www.nytimes.com/2015/09/21/business/a-huge-overnight-increase-in-a-drugs-price-raises-protests.html

Pollin, R., J. Heintz, J., P. Arno, J. Wicks-Lim, and M. Ash. November 30, 2018. "Economic Analysis of Medicare for All." Retrieved from Political Economic Research Institute: https://www.peri.umass.edu/publication/item/1127-economic-analysis-of-medicare-for-all

Porter, M. E., and T. H. Lee. October 2013. "The Strategy That Will Fix Health Care." Retrieved from *Harvard Business Review*: https://hbr.org/2013/10/the-strategy-that-will-fix-health-care

Pramuk, J. February 19, 2019. "House Democrats Unveil a Sweeping 'Medicare-for-All' Bill: Here's What's in It." Retrieved from CNBC: https://www.cnbc.com/2019/02/27/democrat-pramila-jayapal-introduces-medicare-for-all-health-care-bill.html

Ridic, G., S. Gleason, and O. Ridic. 2012. "Comparisons of Health Care Systems in the United States, Germany and Canada." *Materia Sociomedica* 24(2), 112-120. doi:10.5455/msm.2012.24.112-120

Rosenberg, Y. March 22, 2018. "Elizabeth Warren Has a New Plan to Improve Health Care—and It Isn't Medicare for All." Retrieved from *The Fiscal Times*: https://www.thefiscaltimes.com/2018/03/22/Elizabeth-Warren-Has-New-Plan-Improve-Health-Care-and-It-Isn-t-Medicare-All

Rosenthal, Elisabeth. 2017. *An American Sickness: How Healthcare Became Big Business and How You Can Take It Back*. New York: Penguin Books.

Roy, A. December 12, 2014. "Six Reasons Why Vermont's Single-Payer Health Plan Was Doomed from the Start." Retrieved from *Forbes*: https://www.forbesNPR/2014/12/21/6-reasons-why-vermonts-single-payer-health-plan-was-doomed-from-the-start/#265745da4850

Saltzman, E., and C. Eibner. September 2016. "Donald Trump's Health Care Reform Proposals: Anticipated Effects on Insurance Coverage, Out-of-Pocket Costs and the Federal Deficit." Retrieved from the Commonwealth Fund: https://www.commonwealthfund.org/sites/default/files/documents/____media_files_publications_issue_brief_2016_sep_1903_saltzman_trump_hlt_care_reform_proposals_ib_v2.pdf

Sanders, B. 2018. "Options to Finance Medicare for All." Retrieved from Bernie Sanders, Senator: https://www.sanders.senate.gov/download/options-to-finance-medicare-for-all?inline=file

Sanger-Katz, M. February 5, 2017. "Grading Obamacare: Successes, Failures and 'Incompletes.'" Retrieved from *New York Times*: https://www.nytimes.com/2017/02/05/upshot/grading-obamacare-successes-failures-and-incompletes.html

Sass, N. February 26, 2013. "REACT: Bitter Pill: Why Medical Bills Are Killing Us." Retrieved from *The Dinner Table*: https://thedinnertableblog.wordpress.com/2013/02/26/react-bitter-pill-why-medical-bills-are-killing-us-steven-brill-time-magazine/

Schneider, E. C., D. O. Sarnak, D. Squires, A. Shah, and M. M. Doty. July 2017. "Mirror, Mirror 2017: International Comparison Reflects Flaws and Opportunities for Better Healthcare."

Retrieved from the Commonwealth Fund: https://interactives. commonwealthfund.org/2017/july/mirror-mirror/

Scott, D. July 26, 2017. "The Latest Vote to Repeal Obamacare Fails in the Senate." Retrieved from Vox: https://www. vox.com/policy-and-politics/2017/7/26/16034020/ senate-health-care-bill-clean-obamacare-repeal-fails

Seegert, L. November 15, 2017. "U.S. Ranks Worse in Elder Care vs. Other Wealthy Nations." Retrieved from Association of Health Care Journalists: https://healthjournalism.org/ blog/2017/11/u-s-ranks-worse-in-elder-care-vs-other-wealthy-nations/

Selberg, J., B. Sawyer, C. Cox, M. Ramirez, G. Claxton, and L. Levitt. December 6, 2018. "A Generation of Healthcare in the United States: Has Value Improved in the Last 25 Years?" Retrieved from Peterson-Kaiser Health System Tracker: https://www. healthsystemtracker.org/brief/a-generation-of-healthcare-in-the-united-states-has-value-improved-in-the-last-25-years/#item-start

Shen, M. J., and J. P. LaBouff. 2016. "More than Political Ideology: Subtle Racial Prejudice as a Predictor of Opposition to Universal Health Care Among U.S. Citizens." *Journal of Social and Political Psychology* (2), 493–520.

Shi, L., and D. A. Singh. 1998. *Delivering Health Care in America: A Systems Approach*. Gaithersburg, MD: Aspen Publishers.

Singhal, Shubham, Brian Latko, and Carlos Pardo Martin. January 2018. "The Future of Healthcare: Finding the Opportunities that Lie Beneath the Uncertainty." McKinsey & Co. Retrieved from https://www.mckinsey.com

Skocpol, T. Spring 1995. "The Rise and Resounding Demise of the Clinton Plan." *Health Affairs* 14(1), 66–85. doi:10.1377/hlthaff.14.1.66

Soffen, K. September 25, 2017. "There's One Obamacare Repeal Bill Left Standing. Here's What's In It." Retrieved from *Washington Post*: https://www.washingtonpost.com/graphics/2017/politics/cassidy-graham-explainer/?noredirect=on&utm_term=.e8195fdb8727

Spector, J. January 8, 2019. "How New York City Will Provide Health Care to All City Residents." Retrieved from the *Journal News* (lohud.com): https://www.lohud.com/story/news/politics/politics-on-the-hudson/2019/01/08/how-new-york-city-provide-health-care-all-city-residents/2511988002/

Steil, D. July 11, 2018. "The Problem with Employer-Sponsored Insurance." Retrieved from Business Initiative for Health Policy: https://businessinitiative.org/the-problem-with-employer-sponsored-insurance/

Stein, Jeff. April 12, 2019. "'We've Done a Lot More than You Would Think': How the Health-Insurance Industry is Working to Pull Democrats away from Medicare-for-All." Retrieved from *Washington Post*: https://www.washingtonpost.com/business/2019/04/12/weve-done-lot-more-than-you-would-think-how-health-insurance-industry-is-working-pull-democrats-away-medicare-for-all/?noredirect=on&utm_term=.9c61b3ba452c

Sullivan, K. February 26, 2018. "Why Do We Need ACOs and Insurance Companies?" Retrieved from *The Health Care Blog*:

https://thehealthcareblog.com/blog/2018/02/26/why-do-we-need-acos-and-insurance-companies/

Sullivan, P. January 13, 2019. "Booker Tries to Shake Doubts about Pharmaceutical Ties Ahead of 2020." Retrieved from *The Hill*: https://thehill.com/homenews/campaign/424993-booker-tries-to-shake-doubts-about-pharmaceutical-ties-ahead-of-2020

Tao, D. November 29, 2017. "My Army Service Made Me Believe in Universal Health Care." Retrieved from *The Atlantic*: https://www.theatlantic.com/politics/archive/2017/11/my-army-service-made-me-believe-in-universal-health-care/546974/

Tobias, M. September 20, 2017. "Comparing Administrative Costs for Private Insurance and Medicare." Retrieved from Politifact: https://www.politifact.com/truth-o-meter/statements/2017/sep/20/bernie-s/comparing-administrative-costs-private-insurance-a/

Thompson, G. December 3, 2018. "Great Expectations: California's First Steps toward Universal Health Care." Retrieved from Capital & Main: https://capitalandmain.com/californias-first-steps-toward-universal-health-care-1204

Thorlby, R., and S. Arora. 2017. "The English Health Care System." Retrieved from the Commonwealth Fund: https://international.commonwealthfund.org/countries/england/

Tozzi, J., and E. Wasson. March 26, 2019. "Trump Turns Back to Health Care, but What Comes Next Is Unclear." Retrieved from Bloomberg: https://www.bloomberg.com/news/articles/2019-03-26/trump-agencies-won-t-say-what-they-ll-do-if-courts-nix-obamacare

U.S. PIRG. 2018. "Make Health Care Work Better for America."
Retrieved from United States Public Interest Research Group:
https://uspirg.org/issues/usp/make-health-care-work-better-
america

VerValin, J. July 13, 2017. "The Rise and Fall of Vermont's Single
Payer Plan." Retrieved from Cornell Policy Review: http://www.
cornellpolicyreview.com/rise-fall-vermonts-single-payer-plan/

Wallace, J., and Song, Z. 2016. "Traditional Medicare versus Private
Insurance: How Spending, Volume, and Price Change at Age
Sixty-Five." Health Affairs (Project Hope), 35(5), 864–872.
https://doi-org.libproxy.txstate.edu/10.1377/hlthaff.2015.1195

"What Is Value-Based Healthcare?" January 1, 2017. Retrieved from
NEJM Catalyst: https://catalyst.nejm.org/what-is-value-based-
healthcare/

"What Marketplace Health Insurance Plans Cover." 2016. Retrieved
from Healthcare.gov: https://www.healthcare.gov/coverage/
what-marketplace-plans-cover/

Woolhandler, S., D. U. Himmelstein, and A. Gaffney. August 10,
2018. "Single Payer Is Actually a Huge Bargain." Retrieved from
The Nation: https://www.thenation.com/article/single-payer-
actually-huge-bargain/

Yates, R. 2009. "Viewpoint." The Lancet 373, 2078–2081.

Richard George Boudreau is a maxillofacial surgeon, bioethicist, attorney, and forensic expert who serves on the faculty at Loyola-Marymount Univ. Bioethics Institute and Univ. of Calif. Los Angeles Dept. Oral & Maxillofacial Surgery. His quest for education continued unabated since graduating from Univ. of Southern Calif. Dental School and Univ. of Washington, Seattle, Oral & Maxillofacial Surgery Residency. His extensive academic credentials include BS, MA, MBA, DDS, MD, JD, PhD, PsyD degrees and several fellowships. He has dutifully and tirelessly volunteered in several academic teaching capacities and committees over many years and has passionate interests in health care, law, theology, philosophy, education, public policy. He especially enjoys analyzing challenging bioethical issues, authoring articles and books, researching and teaching this scholarly and profound discipline. He is a prolific bioethics lecturer, author, columnist with regular media contributions. One of his alma maters, Pepperdine Univ., honored him in 2011 with the 'George Award' which is awarded to recipients who "exemplify integrity, stewardship, courage, and compassion, while enriching the ever changing world through superior skills and spirit."